Biosensing and Bioimaging: Trends and Perspective

Biosensing and Bioimaging: Trends and Perspective

Editors

Xuemei Wang
Hui Jiang

MDPI • Basel • Beijing • Wuhan • Barcelona • Belgrade • Manchester • Tokyo • Cluj • Tianjin

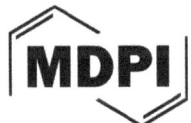

Editors
Xuemei Wang
Southeast University
China

Hui Jiang
Southeast University
China

Editorial Office
MDPI
St. Alban-Anlage 66
4052 Basel, Switzerland

This is a reprint of articles from the Special Issue published online in the open access journal *Biosensors* (ISSN 2079-6374) (available at: https://www.mdpi.com/journal/biosensors/special_issues/Biosensing_Bioimaging).

For citation purposes, cite each article independently as indicated on the article page online and as indicated below:

LastName, A.A.; LastName, B.B.; LastName, C.C. Article Title. *Journal Name* **Year**, *Volume Number*, Page Range.

ISBN 978-3-0365-3973-7 (Hbk)
ISBN 978-3-0365-3974-4 (PDF)

© 2022 by the authors. Articles in this book are Open Access and distributed under the Creative Commons Attribution (CC BY) license, which allows users to download, copy and build upon published articles, as long as the author and publisher are properly credited, which ensures maximum dissemination and a wider impact of our publications.

The book as a whole is distributed by MDPI under the terms and conditions of the Creative Commons license CC BY-NC-ND.

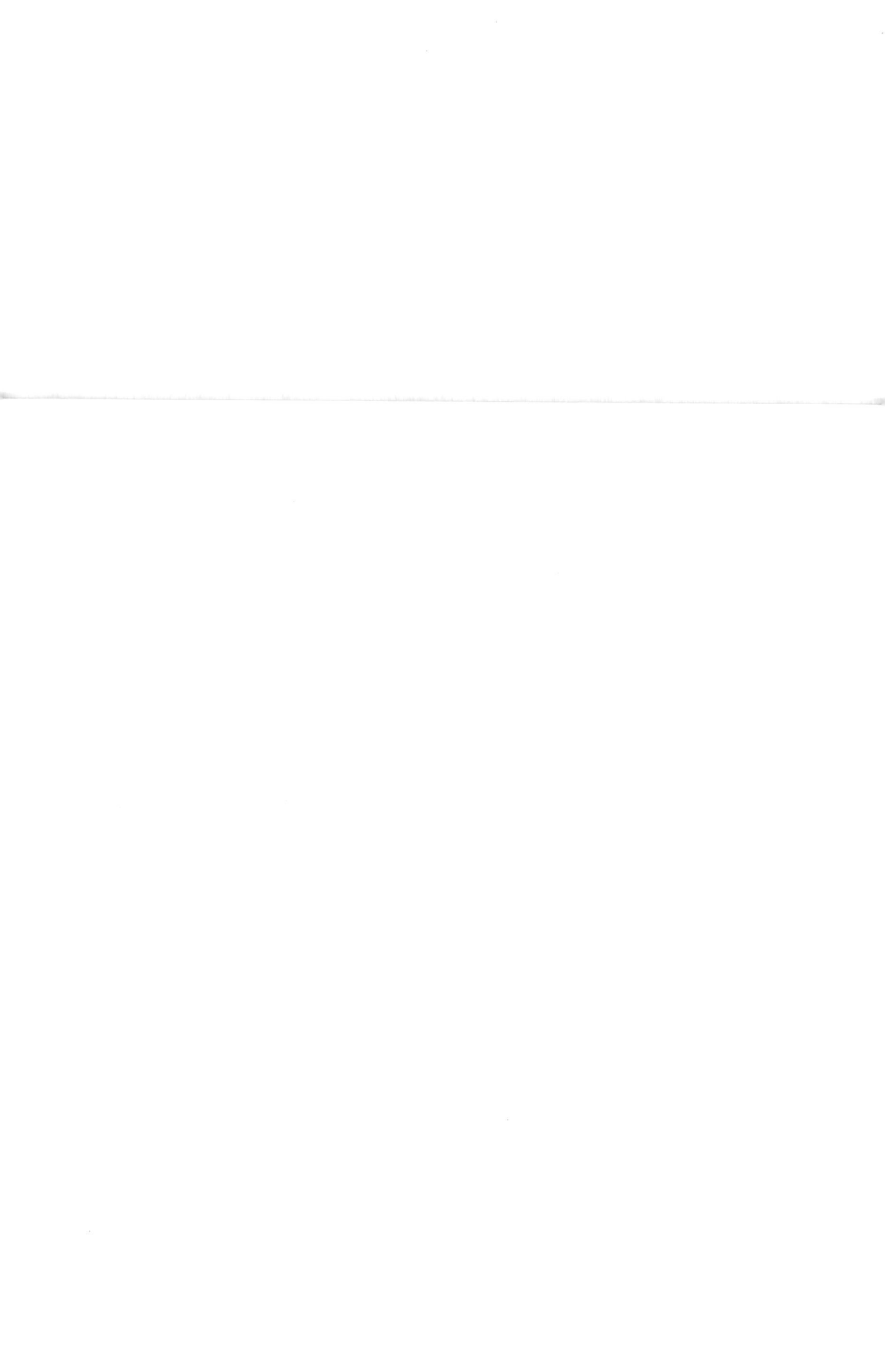

Contents

Preface to "Biosensing and Bioimaging: Trends and Perspective" vii

Weijuan Cai, Liang Yin, Hui Jiang, Yossi Weizmann and Xuemei Wang
Intelligent Bio-Responsive Fluorescent Au–shRNA Complexes for Regulated Autophagy and Effective Cancer Bioimaging and Therapeutics
Reprinted from: *Biosensors* **2021**, *11*, 425, doi:10.3390/bios11110425 1

Jinfeng Quan, Yihan Wang, Jialei Zhang, Kejing Huang, Xuemei Wang and Hui Jiang
Aptamer Embedded Arch-Cruciform DNA Assemblies on 2-D VS_2 Scaffolds for Sensitive Detection of Breast Cancer Cells
Reprinted from: *Biosensors* **2021**, *11*, 378, doi:10.3390/bios11100378 19

Paola Alejandra Fiorani Celedon, Leonardo Maia Leony, Ueriton Dias Oliveira, Natália Erdens Maron Freitas, Ângelo Antônio Oliveira Silva, Ramona Tavares Daltro, Emily Ferreira Santos, Marco Aurélio Krieger, Nilson Ivo Tonin Zanchin and Fred Luciano Neves Santos
Stability Assessment of Four Chimeric Proteins for Human Chagas Disease Immunodiagnosis
Reprinted from: *Biosensors* **2021**, *11*, 289, doi:10.3390/bios11080289 33

Shuang Ding, Haijun Zhang and Xuemei Wang
Microfluidic-Chip-Integrated Biosensors for Lung Disease Models
Reprinted from: *Biosensors* **2021**, *11*, 456, doi:10.3390/bios11110456 47

Xiangdong Lai, Hui Jiang and Xuemei Wang
Biodegradable Metal Organic Frameworks for Multimodal Imaging and Targeting Theranostics
Reprinted from: *Biosensors* **2021**, *11*, 299, doi:10.3390/bios11090299 67

Preface to "Biosensing and Bioimaging: Trends and Perspective"

In recent decades, bioimaging and biosensing have emerged as active research areas that have attracted a tremendous amount of attention in various fields devoted to the visualization of dynamic biological processes and to the in-depth understanding of important disease mechanisms, particularly in precise theranostics and in the effective treatment of intractable diseases, such as cancers. The development of novel bio-responsive material-based biosensors and intelligent supramolecules, or nanoscale probes, has facilitated target bioimaging and smart nano-medicine. Substantial interest has been focused on their versatile roles as excellent biosensing elements and high-resolution contrast agents for multimodal imaging, on the basis of luminescence, magnetics, plasmonics, and high X-ray attenuation properties, among others.

This collection of research articles and reviews in this Special Issue aims to highlight the proceedings in smart biomolecules and nanostructure-based probes for bioimaging and biosensing applications. The topics include intelligent fluorescent shRNA, DNA assembly, chimeric proteins and biodegradable materials. These elements allow electrochemical biosensors, microfluidic chips and multimodal bioimaging systems with high performances to be developed.

We sincerely thank all the editors for the section "Biosensors and Healthcare", published in Biosensors, for their help, and hope that the collection can provide a unique perspective of current biosensing and bioimaging fields.

Xuemei Wang and Hui Jiang
Editors

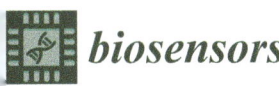

Article

Intelligent Bio-Responsive Fluorescent Au–shRNA Complexes for Regulated Autophagy and Effective Cancer Bioimaging and Therapeutics

Weijuan Cai [1], Liang Yin [2], Hui Jiang [1], Yossi Weizmann [3,*] and Xuemei Wang [1,*]

1. State Key Laboratory of Bioelectronics (Chien-Shiung Wu Lab), School of Biological Science and Medical Engineering, Southeast University, Nanjing 210096, China; 230188127@seu.edu.cn (W.C.); sungj@seu.edu.cn (H.J.)
2. Department of Endocrinology and Metabolism, Shunde Hospital of Southern Medical University, Shunde 528300, China; yinliang151@sina.com
3. Department of Chemistry, Ben-Gurion University of the Negev, Beer-Sheva 8410501, Israel
* Correspondence: yweizmann@bgu.ac.il (Y.W.); xuewang@seu.edu.cn (X.W.)

Abstract: The long non-coding RNA (lncRNA) MALAT1 acts as an oncogene. RNA interference (RNAi) is an effective method to control the expression of specific genes and can be used for the treatment of tumors, but an effective and safe carrier system is a significant obstacle to gene therapy. Herein, we explored the possibility of constructing an in situ bio-responsive self-assembled fluorescent gold-short hairpin RNA nanocomplex (Au–shRNA NCs) delivery system by co-incubating gold and MALAT1-shRNA for precise hepatocellular carcinoma (HCC) imaging and treatment. Due to the characteristics of the cancer microenvironment, Au–shRNA NCs self-assembled in HCC cells (HepG2) but did not occur in control cells (L02) under the same conditions. The in situ bio-responsive self-assembled Au–shRNA NCs delivery system can realize cancer cell bioimaging and promote cell uptake and endosomal escape mechanism, thereby realizing effective transfection. They effectively silenced target gene MALAT1, and with the downregulation of MALAT1, we found that several molecules involved in autophagic flux were also regulated. In vitro and tumor-bearing mouse model experiments demonstrated that the as-prepared fluorescent Au–shRNA NCs can readily realize tumor bioimaging and effectively silence the target gene MALAT1, and those autophagy-related pathway molecules were significantly downregulated, thereby exerting a tumor suppressor efficiency. This raises the possibility of realizing accurate multi-scale bio-imaging from the molecular-level with targeted gene-recognition to cancer cell imaging as well as in vivo tumor tissue imaging for the simultaneous precise cancer therapy.

Keywords: bio-responsive fluorescent complexes; shRNA delivery; LncRNA MALAT1; cancer cells bioimaging; therapeutics; autophagy

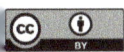

1. Introduction

Long noncoding RNAs (lncRNAs) are more than 200 nucleotides in length [1,2] and participate in numerous physiological and pathophysiological activities such as carcinogenesis and autophagy [3–5]. Aberrant expression or dysfunction of lncRNAs is closely associated with various diseases [6–9]. Recently, research findings have illustrated that lncRNAs may also be involved in remodeling the tumor microenvironment and in tumor metastasis [10]. Metastasis-associated lung adenocarcinoma transcript 1 (MALAT1) is one of the star molecules of lncRNA, which has been determined to participate in various processes including cell apoptosis and proliferation [11]. As reported in several studies, MALAT1 serves as a potentially valuable biomarker in cancer diagnosis and prognosis [12]. Meta-analyses have shown the association between high MALAT1 level and poor clinical outcomes [13,14]. In addition, it is reported that MALAT1 is a mutation factor associated with the occurrence of hepatocellular carcinoma (HCC) [15]. However, how MALAT1 can be used to target HCC therapeutically and the underlying mechanism remain largely unknown.

RNA interference (RNAi) is considered to be a gene silencing phenomenon present in most eukaryotic cells. RNAi has the potential to treat almost any disease by using appropriate sequences to silence the expression of virtually any target gene [16]. Small interfering RNAs (siRNAs) are effector molecules in the process of RNAi [17]. Although the simplest RNAi method is cytoplasmic delivery via siRNA oligonucleotides, the technology is restricted to cells suitable for transfection and is mainly used in transient expression study. An exogenously introduced expressing short hairpin RNA (shRNA) has similar functions to siRNA and can also exert RNAi effects [18]. The shRNA can be converted into siRNA in the cell to exert a gene silencing effect and achieve long-term knockdown of the targeted gene. In addition, shRNA is being rapidly developed into a new avenue for gene function analysis and a new treatment modality. However, this approach faces significant challenges in achieving tissue specificity and the safe and effective delivery of shRNA.

Several obstacles related to systemic shRNA delivery include clearance by the reticuloendothelial system, the complex extracellular matrix and environment around tumor cells, off-target effects, and poor cellular uptake [19,20]. Given the above, in this study, we designed in situ bio-self-assembled Au–shRNA nanocomplexes (Au–shRNA NCs), then examined their ability to silence target gene MALAT1 and their effectiveness in tumor bioimaging and treatment. Currently, the alarming incidence of chronic hepatitis B virus and C has led to most HCCs, and these cases have become the third leading cause of cancer death [21,22]. HCC has been mechanistically explored in some studies, but these efforts have not improved survival. Thus, it is vital to exploit the molecular mechanisms that regulate the metastatic behavior of HCC to develop new therapies that target HCC. More importantly, this approach can also accurately help real-time tumor monitoring and bioimaging. MALAT1 has unique mechanisms of action in different types of cancer [23], which acts as an oncogenic lncRNA in HCC and is often highly expressed [24,25]. Autophagy is a conservative lysosome-mediated intracellular catabolic process, which is very important for cellular homeostasis [26]. Studies have shown that lncRNA plays a crucial role in the process of autophagy [27]. MALAT1 promotes proliferation and metastasis of invasive pancreatic cancer through autophagy stimulation [28]. Silencing MALAT1 can inhibit chemically induced autophagy, while overexpression of MALAT1 can promote autophagy in gastric cancer [11]. However, whether silencing MALAT1 affects HCC cell autophagy is unclear.

The bioimaging process is the most direct and effective way for biological structure and function research. It uses optical or electron microscopes to directly obtain microstructure images of biological cells and/or tissues, and understands various physiological processes of biological cells through the analysis of the resulting images [29]. Furthermore, applying new materials such as nanomaterials makes imaging technology play a more significant role [30]. At present, the growing trend of bioimaging technology also requires the advancing direction of molecular imaging technology not only for clinical diagnosis and treatment, but also for new drug development and basic research of human science.

Herein, we explored a new approach of the systemic shRNA delivery for lncRNA MALAT1-regulated autophagy via the in situ synthesis of bio-self-assembled Au–shRNA NCs in HCC cells/or in vivo tissues. Biological imaging techniques such as confocal, transmission electron microscopy (TEM), and atomic force microscopy (AFM) help us observe that the ability of the as-prepared fluorescent Au–shRNA NCs to regulate target gene MALAT1 on autophagy and silence MALAT1, and demonstrate its efficiency for the real-time imaging and monitoring of tumor treatments. This raises the possibility of the in vivo utilization of this novel Au–shRNA NC delivery system via RNAi to inhibit HCC progression and realize effective HCC imaging and therapy.

2. Materials and Methods

2.1. Cell Culture

In the research, we purchased human hepatocarcinoma cell lines (HepG2, SMMC-7721) and control cells (human embryonic liver L02) from ATCC (Manassas, VA, USA). L02, HepG2, and SMMC-7721 cells were cultured with DMEM (4.5 g/L glucose) supplemented with 1% penicillin/streptomycin and 10% fetal bovine serum (all from Gibco, Australia). The culture conditions were strictly at 37 °C, 5% CO_2, and a 95% humidity environment.

2.2. Patients and Specimens

This study was approved by the First Affiliated Hospital, Shihezi University School of Medicine. From May 2019 to January 2021, a total of 30 tumor tissues and matched normal adjacent tissues were collected from HCC patients registered to our hospital through surgical resection. Importantly, all tissues were snap-frozen in liquid nitrogen until further use. We excluded patients from receiving chemotherapy or radiotherapy preoperatively or postoperatively. All human samples were obtained with the patients' written consent. In Table S1, the clinicopathological characteristics of the HCC patients are listed in detail.

2.3. qRT-PCR

We used TRIzol reagent (Invitrogen, USA) to isolate the total RNA from frozen tissue. Before further experiments, the purity and concentration of the extracted RNA samples were quantified using NanoDrop ND-1000 equipment. The steps described in the Hairpin-it qRT-PCR Kit (GenePharma Co., Shanghai, China) were followed to reverse-transcribe the total RNA (2 μg) of each sample. Then, the qRT-PCR ran according to the qRT-PCR Kit instructions, and the CT values were obtained after the end of the reaction. Finally, the relative changes in gene expression were calculated by the $2^{-\Delta\Delta CT}$ method. In this experiment, GAPDH was used as an internal control. The primer sequences were purchased from Invitrogen (Waltham, MA, USA) and are shown in Table S2. All PCR runs were performed in triplicate.

2.4. MTT Cytotoxicity Assessment and Cytostatic Test

Initially, deionized water was used to dilute the $HAuCl_4$ (Shanghai Yuanye Bio, China, CAS:27988-77-8, pH = 7.2) to create solutions with the appropriate concentrations for the toxicity tests. Briefly, we took the prepared liquid with a concentration of 10 nM $HAuCl_4$, and then diluted it according to the experimental design. The final concentration gradient was 0, 0.5, 1, 5, 10, 30, 50, 100, 200, and 500 μM for the experiment. Then, we used trypsin to digest L02 and HepG2 cells, and 200 μL complete medium containing approximately 4000 cells was placed in 96-well plates. Following this, the experimental arrangement was incubated with different concentrations of $HAuCl_4$ for 48 h and the experiment proceeded following instructions in the MTT Kit where the absorbance measurement needs to be performed at a wavelength of 490 nm. Next, according to the concentration range provided in the instructions, the best shRNA concentration and silencing effect were determined. Finally, HepG2 cells in the logarithmic growth phase were seeded in a single cell suspension in a 96-well plate, and a cytostatic test was carried out for five days. After 24 h of incubation, complete fresh medium was added to the cells, followed by the addition of $HAuCl_4$ and shRNA1 successively, and then co-incubated for 0, 1, 2, 3, 4, and 5 days. The concentrations of shRNA1 and $HAuCl_4$ were 3 ng/μL and 5 μM, respectively. At each time interval point, we analyzed the absorbance value and drew the cell growth curve. Each experiment needed to ensure that three biological replicates were used.

2.5. Wound Healing Assay

A 6-well plate to culture cells was used (the number of cells per well is the same), and when the cell density reached 80–90%, a p200 pipette tip was employed to scrape the cells. Different groups of cells at 0, 12, 24, and 48 h were processed, and their images were captured at the same time interval, respectively. Finally, all images were analyzed using

ImageJ software. In this experiment, the concentrations of shRNA1 and HAuCl$_4$ were 3 ng/µL and 5 µM in the Au–shRNA1 NC group, respectively.

2.6. In Situ Biosynthetic Au–shRNA1 NCs

Adherent HepG2 cells in culture were exposed to HAuCl$_4$ solution at a final concentration of 5 µM. The cells were gently shaken to mix the solution well with the medium. Then, the cells were put back into the cell incubator. After a few minutes, the cells were settled, and the shRNA1 plasmid (ViGene Biosciences, China) that silences MALAT1 was added to the medium for co-incubation. After incubating for at least 24 h, the medium was first discarded. Next, the cells were washed three times with PBS and trypsinized for 1–2 min. The remaining trypsin solution was removed, and 2 mL PBS was added, and the sample was centrifuged in a sterile centrifuge at 1500 rpm for 3 min. After that, the supernatant was removed, and deionized water was added to resuspend the cells. As previously described [31], the repeated freeze–thaw method was used to prepare the cell extracts for further characterization.

2.7. Cellular Uptake and Colocalization Studies

HepG2 cells were plated (1 × 10^6 cells per well) on a laser confocal culture dish, and the cells were first pretreated with various endocytosis inhibitors for about 1 h, then, gold salt and shRNA were added sequentially and incubated with the cells for 6 h. The concentrations of the inhibitors was as follows: 37 mg/mL methyl-β-cyclodextrin, 10 µg/mL chlorpromazine, 10 mg/mL rottlerin, 200 µg/mL genistein, and 5 µg/mL filipin III (Sigma-Aldrich, MO, USA). After 6 h of co-incubation, the HepG2 cells were washed three times with PBS and fixed with 4% paraformaldehyde for 30 min. The cell nucleus was stained with DAPI (Beyotime, Shanghai, China). Finally, a confocal microscope was used to image the sample with 488 nm (Leica, Wetzlar, Germany).

To observe the subcellular localization of Au–shRNA NCs, gold salt and the shRNA were co-incubated with HepG2 cells at 37 °C for 12 h. The specific experimental process was the same as that above-mentioned. Endosomes and lysosomes were labeled by Lysotracker Red for 30 min and washed with PBS (three times), followed by nuclei staining with DAPI for 3 min. The images were obtained by confocal microscopy (Leica, Wetzlar, Germany).

2.8. Transmission Electron Microscopy (TEM)

We first diluted the Au–shRNA1 NC extracts with deionized water, then dropped it on the copper grid and waited for it to dry naturally. We used TEM (JEM-2100, JEOL Ltd., Tokyo, Japan) to characterize the size and distribution confirmation of the in situ formation of Au–shRNA1 NCs. In addition, we also evaluated the structure of lysosomes and autophagosomes and/or autolysosomes through bio-TEM. Briefly, HepG2 cells were seeded in 6-well plates and processed according to different groups. After 24 h of incubation, the cells were collected, the culture medium was discarded, and the electron microscope fixation solution (glutaraldehyde) was added for fixation. Finally, the cells were observed under TEM (Hitachi-HT7700, Hitachi High-Tech Corporation, Tokyo, Japan) and collected for image analysis.

2.9. Atomic Force Microscopy (AFM)

Before adding the sample, the mica flakes (15 mm × 15 mm) were immersed in Mg^{2+} solution (10 nM MgCl$_2$ solution) for 5 min in advance. Next, the lysis sample (10 µL) with deionized water was deposited onto freshly cleaved mica to adsorb for 5 min, rinsed gently with distilled water, and then we waited for a few minutes until the specimen was dry. The morphology and characteristics of Au–shRNA1 NCs were characterized by AFM (Bruker Dimension Icon, Bruker, Billerica, MA, USA). The concentrations of shRNA1 and HAuCl$_4$ added to the original extraction solution were 3 ng/µL and 5 µM, respectively.

2.10. Fluorescence Confocal Microscopy

HepG2 cells were seeded on a laser confocal culture dish, processed according to different groups, and incubated for 24–48 h. Next, HepG2 cells were fixed (4% paraformaldehyde) for 30 min, washed with PBS three times, and then permeabilized with 0.3% Triton X-100 for 20 min. Finally, DAPI was added to stain the HepG2 cell nuclei (blue). The images were obtained by confocal microscopy (Leica, Wetzlar, Germany).

2.11. Western Blot Analysis

Western blotting was performed as described previously [31,32]. Briefly, whole-cell lysates containing approximately 40 µg of protein were loaded on 10% sodium dodecyl sulfate-polyacrylamide gel electrophoresis. Then, the transfer of the PVDF membrane was carried out by the electrotransfer method. After that, the membranes were incubated with the antibodies listed in Table S3. According to the experiment, we added the appropriate secondary antibody and incubated it together, then captured the blots on the Bio-Rad chemiluminescence imager. We then used ImageJ software for relative protein content analysis. The experimental internal reference was GAPDH and repeated three times.

2.12. GFP-(Microtubule-Associated Protein 1 Light Chain 3 (LC3)/Lysosomal-Associated Membrane Protein2 (LAMP2)/p62 Staining

Different groups of cells were processed according to the experimental conditions and cultured on laser confocal Petri dishes. After incubation with shRNA1 and gold salt for 24–48 h, HepG2 cells were washed twice with cold 1 × PBS, then placed in the fixative solution (4% paraformaldehyde) for 30 min in the same method as described for the fluorescence confocal microscopy and permeabilized for 20 min. Subsequently, 6.5% bovine serum albumin was added to block the cells for 40 min. Anti-LAMP2/green fluorescent protein-LC3 (GFP-LC3)/p62 antibodies were added for incubation, and then FITC/tetramethylrhodamine-conjugated secondary antibodies were used for fluorescent staining. Cells were stained with DAPI to visualize the nuclei, where the green dots indicate LAMP2 staining, whereas the red dots indicate GFP-LC3/p62 staining. The observed yellow dots, due to the merger of the red and green channels, represent autophagosomes. Finally, immunofluorescence was analyzed under a confocal microscope (Leica TCS SPE, Leica, Wetzlar, Germany). In this experiment, the final concentrations of shRNA1 and HAuCl$_4$ were 3 ng/µL and 5µM, respectively, and the total volume in the laser confocal culture dish was 2 mL.

2.13. Orthotopic Tumor Model

We purchased several four-week-old BALB/c athymic nude mice from SPF (Beijing) Biotechnology Co. Ltd., Beijing, China and established the tumor model to simulate the natural cancer microenvironment. All animals were kept strictly by the standards and followed the guidance of the Southeast University Animal Research Ethics Committee to conduct all experiments involving mice. HepG2 cells (5 × 10^7) in 100 µL PBS were injected into the left side of the mouse abdomen using a sterile syringe (1 mL).

When the tumor reached a diameter of about 3 mm, 16 tumor-bearing mice were randomly subdivided further into four groups, and four different preparations were injected five times intravenously every three days. Normal saline (control, 100 µL), free shRNA1 (40 µg), Au NCs (2 mM HAuCl$_4$, 100 µL), and Au–shRNA1 NCs (2 mM HAuCl$_4$, 100 µL; 40 µg shRNA1) were injected into the four groups (n = 4 mice per group). Then, in vivo fluorescence imaging was performed at 0, 12, 24, and 48 h, and the wavelength of the excitation filter was 460 nm. The mice were anesthetized with 2% isoflurane gas, observed with an IVIS Lumina XRMS Series III (Perkin Elmer, Waltham, MA, USA), and the experimental results were recorded. In addition, the body weight of the mice and tumor volume needed to be measured and observed every three days. At the end of the treatment cycle (day 15), all mice were euthanized. The tumor xenografts were harvested and strictly weighed and the main organs dissected for further analyses. Finally, we detected the levels of autophagy-related molecules in different groups of the tumor xenografts by western blotting.

2.14. Statistical Analysis

In this study, the statistical analysis software used included GraphPad Prism 8.0 and Origin 8.5. We tested the normality and the variance homogeneity of the data, which were shown as mean ± standard deviation (SD). All experiments required three biological replicates. We used the Student's t-test to compare differences between the means of the two groups. Two-way analysis of variance was used to make paired observations and repeat measurements over time. Significance in statistical analysis was defined as $p < 0.05$.

3. Results and Discussion

3.1. Elevated Expression of MALAT1 Identified in HCC Patients and HCC Cell Lines

In recent years, a cancer-specific data repository called Oncomine [33,34] has been created and has been of enormous utility for cancer researchers. The MALAT1 expression in liver cancer was compared with those in normal samples using the Oncomine online database. The list was obtained using a meta-analysis of Oncomine data (Figure S1a). The scoring of MALAT1 overexpression in liver cancer samples (hepatocellular adenoma and HCC, using a set of three studies containing 160 samples) versus normal controls is shown [35,36]. Lnc2Cancer 3.0 is an updated version of the cancer storage system that includes investigational support for human cancer-associated lncRNAs and related data [37]. Lnc2Cancer 3.0 was used to obtain detailed data on MALAT1 in HCC including box plots, stage plots, and survival plots (Figure S1b–d). The relevant observations for MALAT1 in HCC demonstrated higher expression levels of MALAT1 in HCC than the controls ($p < 0.01$). The MALAT1 expression in HCC tumors and corresponding adjacent non-cancer tissues (ANCTs) were evaluated by qRT-PCR. The increased expression level of MALAT1 was observed in HCC samples compared with ANCTs (Figure S1e). Moreover, we found that MALAT1 expression was significantly higher in HepG2 and SMMC-7721 than in L02 (Figure S1f). Next, we analyzed the relationship between MALAT1 expression level and disease progression and prognosis in HCC patients (Table S1). In brief, the above results suggest that MALAT1 might be a high-risk factor for the occurrence and development of HCC.

3.2. In Situ Self-Assembly of Au–shRNA NCs

Based on the above observations, we investigated the possibility of utilizing the specific pathological environment of HCC for the in situ bio-self-assembled Au–shRNA NCs to achieve biological effects (e.g., RNAi) for target cancer theranostics. As we know, due to different pH values, tumor cells/tissues will spontaneously produce a large amount of active substances, which causes the tumor microenvironment to be different from normal tissues [38,39]. The unique characteristics of the tumor microenvironment can be exploited by in situ imaging due to the presence of relatively high amounts of specific agents that can act as reducing agents of gold ions for producing fluorescent Au NCs [40–42]. Similar to those of siRNA, the related bases of shRNA are negatively charged [43]. Thus, positively charged Au(III) salt reduction can readily attach to negatively charged shRNA, leading to efficient shRNA intracellular transfection to construct fluorescent Au–shRNA NCs. Meanwhile, we observed that in the unique microenvironment of cancer cells, the fluorescent Au–shRNA NCs can readily self-assemble to facilitate tumor bioimaging and treatments, especially when realizing precise RNA silencing effects (Figure 1).

3.3. Characterization of Au–shRNA NC Uptake and Escape

To explore possible uptake mechanisms, in this study, we used different inhibitors that inhibit specific endocytic pathways. Methyl-β-cyclodextrin (inhibits lipid-raft-mediated endocytosis), chlorpromazine (inhibits clathrin-mediated endocytosis), rottlerin (inhibits macropinocytosis), genistein (inhibits caveolae-mediated endocytosis pathway), and filipin

III inhibitors were used in our study. We used laser confocal microscopy to image and excited at 488 nm (Figure 2a–f). The effect of different inhibitors on the uptake of Au–shRNA NC by living HepG2 cells was analyzed in detail, as shown in Figure S2. The results demonstrated that the cells treated with rottlerin significantly reduced the uptake of Au–shRNA NCs compared to the control group. Second, the cells treated with methyl-β-cyclodextrin, chloropromazine, and genistein were also reduced to a certain extent compared with the control. This result suggests that these Au–shRNA NCs are internalized predominantly via the macropinocytosis pathway. Meanwhile, this also suggests a significant role of the lipid-raft-mediated pathway in the uptake, and the caveolae-mediated pathway and clathrin-mediated pathway are also involved in the uptake of Au–shRNA NCs by HepG2 cells.

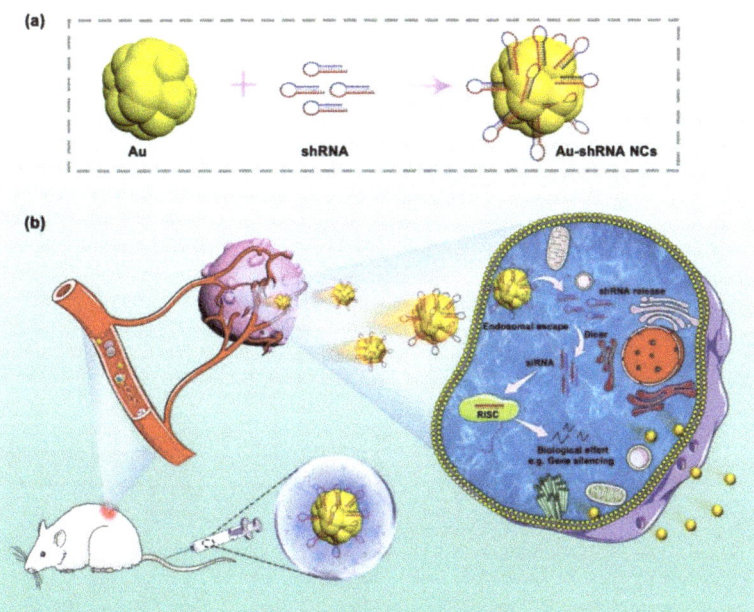

Figure 1. Schematic illustration of the in situ bio-self-assembled fluorescent Au–shRNA NCs to achieve biological effects for cancer imaging and theranostics.

Endosomal escape is another major factor of the intracellular fate of Au–shRNA NCs after successful cell internalization. Complexes entering the cell via one or more endocytic pathway become entrapped in the vesicles, the vesicles mature, forming early endosomes and late endosomes, and eventually end up in the lysosome. The complexes are effective in achieving endosome escape, otherwise, enzymatic degradation processes take place [44]. Therefore, endosomal escape is also very important for shRNA delivery. If these intracellular nanocomplexes cannot escape from the endosome or lysosome, the Au–shRNA NCs cannot release the encapsulated shRNA into the cytoplasm or nucleus for tumor therapy. Therefore, we further investigated the intracellular distribution and colocalization of Au–shRNA NCs and endosomes/lysosomes by confocal microscopy imaging. Our previous study showed that in situ self-assembly gold nanoclusters in the presence of miRNA/DNA can generate green fluorescence spontaneously at 488 nm [31,32]. Fluorescent cellular images of shRNA and gold salt treated cells (i.e., after co-incubation for 12 h) are shown in Figure 2g. Through imaging, it can be seen that most of the bio-self-assembly Au–shRNA NCs escaped from the endosomes/lysosomes, while the rest were captured, preventing their accumulation in the cytoplasm, which are shown as yellow dots in the image. The position and number of protonable free tertiary amine groups in Au–shRNA NCs may promote the retention of this small part of the nanocomposite [44]. Taken together, with the help of confocal imaging, we intuitively observed that the self-assembled Au–shRNA NC delivery system can successfully realize cellular internalization in targeted cancer cells, and have better endosomal escape capabilities in HepG2 cells.

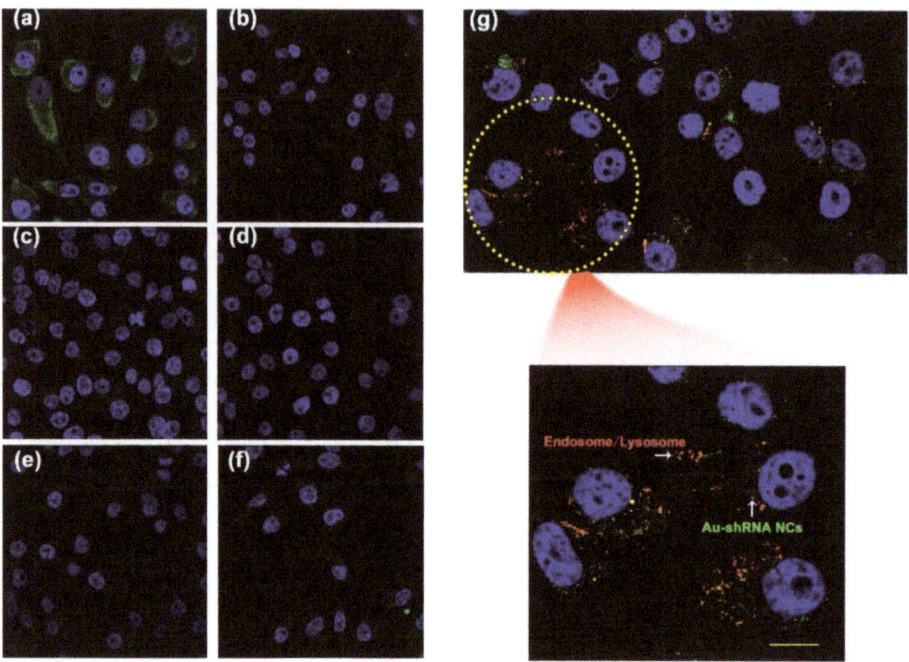

Figure 2. Characterization of Au–shRNA NC uptake and escape. Effect of inhibitors on the uptake of Au–shRNA NCs by live HepG2 cells. When excited at 488 nm, fluorescent confocal images of cells after incubation with Au–shRNA NCs in the absence (**a**) and presence of methyl-β-cyclodextrin (**b**), chloropromazine (**c**), rottlerin (**d**), genistein (**e**), and filipin III (**f**). 4′,6-Diamino-2-phenylindole (DAPI) was used for nucleic staining. (**g**) Colocalization between Au–shRNA1 NCs and endosomes/lysosomes. Green: Au–shRNA1 NCs by 488 nm excitation, Blue: nucleus stained by DAPI; Red: lysosome stained by Lysotracker Red. Scale bar: 10 µm.

3.4. Effective Silencing of Target Gene MALAT1 via Au–shRNA NCs

To demonstrate the feasibility of the synthesized Au–shRNA NCs to silence MALAT1 in HCCs, we first performed cytotoxicity testing on L02 and HepG2 cells. These results indicate that gold salt ($HAuCl_4$ solution) has outstanding biocompatibility with HepG2 and L02 cells. For HepG2 cells, after 48 h of incubation in $HAuCl_4$ with a final concentration of ≤5 µM, cell viability remained greater than 80% (Figure 3a). Based on these observations, we further examined the ability of shRNA1 and shRNA2 to silence MALAT1 in HepG2 cells by incubating the cells with gold salt. According to the instructions, we constructed two optimized concentrations of shRNA (1.5 ng/µL, 3.0 ng/µL). The most obviously silencing effect on MALAT1 was at the concentration of shRNA1 (3.0 ng/µL) (Figure 3b). Analysis of the in situ gold nanotransfection shRNA-mediated inhibition indicated that not only was the effect in the presence of $HAuCl_4$ notably higher than that without $HAuCl_4$, but the effect of shRNA1 with $HAuCl_4$ solution was also better than that of shRNA2 with $HAuCl_4$. In addition, the inhibitory effect at 24 h was obviously lower than that at 48 h (Figure 3c). Moreover, we examined the ability of shRNA1 and shRNA2 at concentrations of 3.0 ng/µL to silence MALAT1 in HCC cells by the Lipofectamine 3000 Transfection Reagent

(Invitrogen, USA, Lip 3000) (Figure 3d). Consistent with the above results, shRNA1 was better than shRNA2 in silencing MALAT1 by Lip 3000. Thus, shRNA1 was selected for MALAT1 silencing in subsequent experiments at a concentration of 3.0 ng/μL.

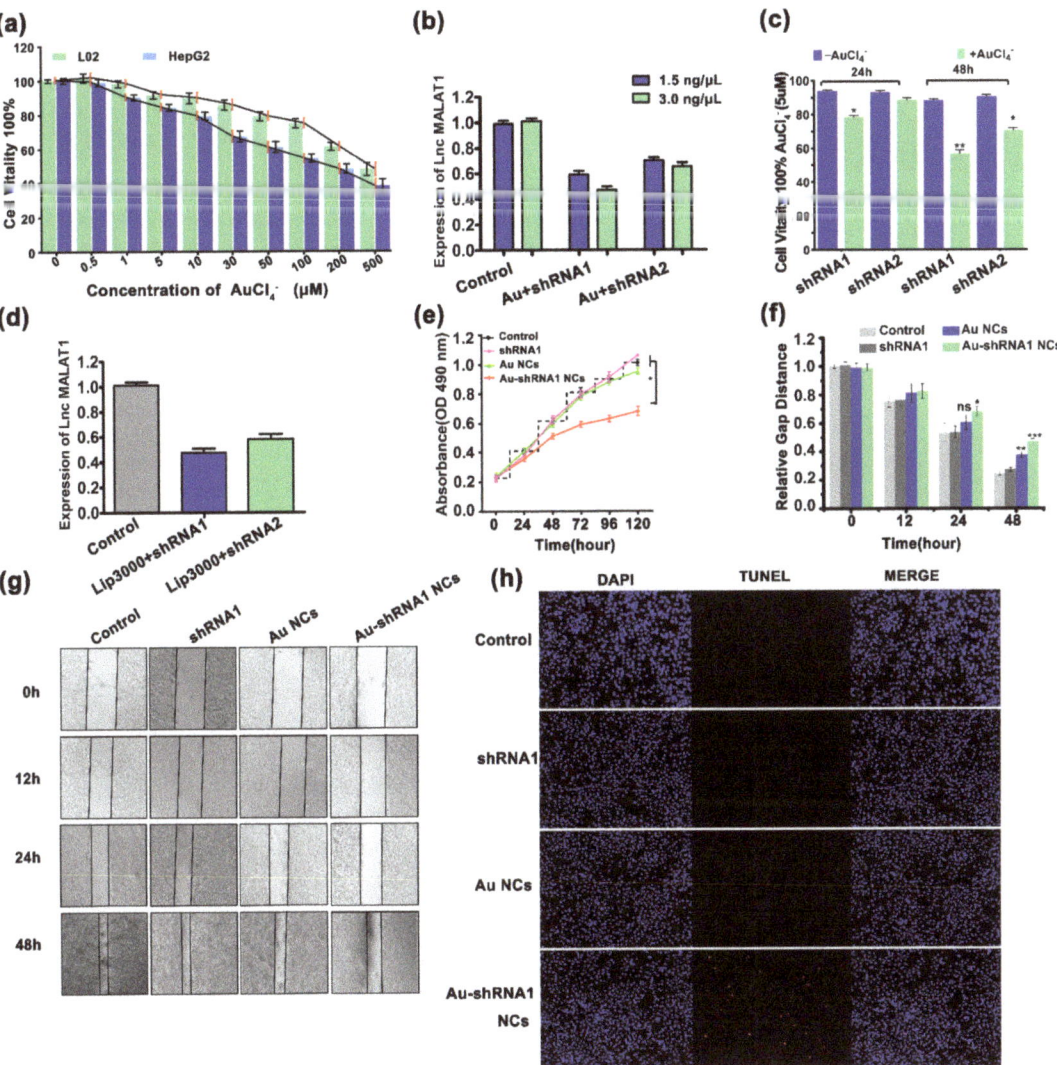

Figure 3. Biochemical characteristics of bio-self-assembled Au–shRNA NCs. (**a**) MTT cell viability and toxicity analysis of HepG2 and L02 cells with HAuCl4. (**b**) MTT assay of HepG2 cells with Au–shRNA NCs generated with different concentrations of shRNA1 and shRNA2 (normalized to unprocessed cells). (**c**) The inhibitory effects of shRNA1 and shRNA2 with (green) and without (blue) gold salt in HepG2 cells at 24/48 h treatment. (**d**) The ability of 3 ng/μL shRNA1 and shRNA2 to silence MALAT1 in HepG2 cells was examined by Lip 3000 transfection. (**e**) Long-term (5-day) MTT proliferation analysis of HepG2 cells under different conditions (ANOVA, * $p < 0.05$). Control group (unprocessed), shRNA1 group (shRNA1, 3 ng/μL), Au NCs group (HAuCl4, 5 μM), and Au–shRNA1 NC group (shRNA1, 3 ng/μL; HAuCl4, 5 μM). (**f**,**g**) The corresponding HepG2 cell scratch-healing experimental analysis and morphological images are also displayed. ** $p < 0.01$, *** $p < 0.001$. (**h**) HepG2 cells treated with shRNA1 with or without gold salt were analyzed by the TUNEL assay. The red color indicates cell apoptosis, and the blue color indicates HepG2 cell nucleus.

3.5. Cell Proliferation Inhibition and Apoptosis via Au–shRNA1 NCs

The cell proliferation of the Au–shRNA1 NCs group was significantly lower than that of the non-treatment and Au NC group in the 5-day MTT assay (Figure 3e). Through scratch healing experiments, we found that the migration of HepG2 cells with Au–shRNA1 NCs was significantly decreased (Figure 3f,g). Moreover, the percentage of TUNEL positive nuclei (31.16%) in the Au–shRNA1 NC group was significantly higher than the control (0.66%) and the Au NC (4.66%) group ($p < 0.05$; Figure 3h and Figure S3). These observations demonstrate that the generated bio-responsive self-assembling biosynthetic Au–shRNA1 NCs could enhance apoptosis and retard the migration and proliferation of cancer cells.

3.6. Physicochemical Characteristics of Bio-Self-Assembled Au–shRNA1 NCs

To verify the conformation of Au–shRNA1 NCs, we harvested cytoplasmic extracts from cells and further characterized them by TEM and AFM. The TEM image clearly shows the in situ self-assembly Au–shRNA1 NCs in the HepG2 cell extract (Figure 4a,b). When shRNA1 was added, Au NCs with a diameter of about 2–3 nm were clearly visible. This is consistent with our previous research results on gold nanoclusters in the presence of miRNA/DNA [31,32]. Figure 4c–e shows the AFM images of self-assembled biosynthetic Au–shRNA1 NCs isolated from HepG2 cells that had been incubated with shRNA1 and gold salt. The height analysis of the scribe part of the AFM diagram shows that the cumulative height of Au–shRNA1 NCs appears to be approximately 2–3 nm, and the above result is consistent with the TEM characterization. Moreover, HepG2 cells can spontaneously form fluorescent Au NCs under 488 nm excitation by laser confocal fluorescence microscopy. The existence of self-assembled Au–shRNA1 NCs was successfully indicated by green fluorescence inside the cells, and were well dispersed around the nucleoli of the cells, where DAPI were used to stain the nuclei (Figure 4f). We observed that the intracellular fluorescence intensity of the Au–shRNA1 NCs culture group was higher than that of the gold salt-only culture group. This observation suggests that these Au–shRNA1 NCs can enhance intracellular fluorescence. In contrast, such fluorescent characteristics were not observed in L02 cells under all experimental conditions (Figure S4).

3.7. Inhibition of Autophagic Flux through Silencing of MALAT1 by Au–shRNA1 NCs

Studies suggest that autophagy is associated with poor clinical prognosis of certain cancers, and inhibition of autophagy has been shown to reduce cancer growth [11,28,45]. Biological imaging is an important research method to understand the tissue structure of organisms and clarify various physiological functions of organisms. In the current study, the bio-TEM image was performed to confirm the formation of autophagosomes in different groups. The bio-TEM image shows that the whole cell was a long spindle shape, the edge of the cell membrane was relatively complete, the cell matrix was evenly distributed, and the organelles were abundant. The noticeable difference was that there were fewer autophagosomes in the Au–shRNA NC group compared to the other groups (red arrow). Our findings revealed an obvious decrease in the cytoplasmic structures of autophagosomes and autolysosomes and lysosomes in HepG2 cells after co-incubation with gold salt and the shRNA1 (Figure 5a). Compared with the control group and the Au NC group, the autophagy level of the Au–shRNA1 NC group was reduced. Western blot image analysis also supports this result (Figure 5b,c). In order to explore the correlation between MALAT1 silencing and autophagy flux in HepG2 cells, western blot analysis was performed to detect LC3 to determine the abundance of autophagosomes in the cytoplasm. LC3 is currently recognized as a marker for autophagy [46]. During the formation of autophagy, the cytoplasmic LC3 (i.e., LC3-I) will enzymatically decompose a small segment of the membrane and transform it into (autophagosome) membrane (i.e., LC3-II). The ratio of LC3-II/I can estimate the level of autophagy. p62 can connect LC3 and ubiquitinated substrates, and then be integrated into autophagosomes, and degraded in autophagolysosomes, so it is used as an indicator of autophagy degradation [47]. Therefore, it can be considered that the decrease in the ratio of LC3-II/I and the increase in p62 level during the autophagic flux of organisms indicate autophagy inhibition. LAMP2 is a lysosomal membrane protein that can be used to monitor autophagosome and lysosome fusion. Our results showed that compared with the control group and the Au NC group, the Au–shRNA1 NC group had a significantly lower LC3-II/I level, while the p62 level was significantly increased.

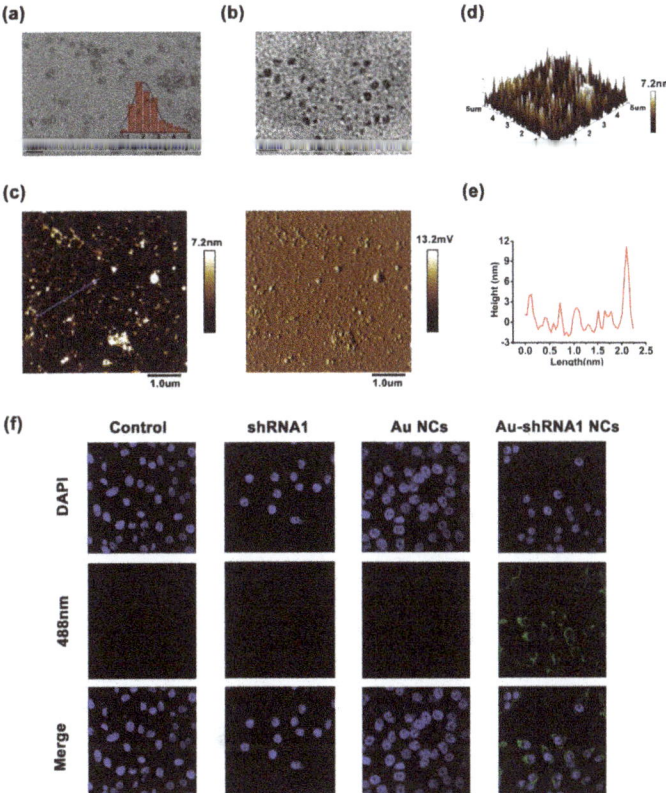

Figure 4. Physicochemical characteristics of bio-self-assembled Au–shRNA1 NCs. (a) Typical TEM and (b) a higher magnification TEM image of Au–shRNA1 NCs obtained from HepG2 cells after 48 h of culture with HAuCl$_4$ (5 µM) and shRNA1 (3 ng/µL). (c) Typical AFM height diagram (**left**) and corresponding phase diagram (**right**) of the isolated Au–shRNA1 NCs. (d) A 3D model diagram corresponding to (c). (e) Height analysis of the underlined area in (c) (**left**). (f) Laser confocal fluorescence images of HepG2 cells cultured with DMEM, the shRNA1, gold salt, or both the shRNA1 and gold salt. After excitement at 488 nm, visualization of biosynthetic fluorescent Au–shRNA1 NCs in HepG2 cells by fluorescence imaging DAPI was used for nucleic staining. In the above tests, the concentration of shRNA1 was 3 ng/µL, while that of HAuCl$_4$ was 5 µM.

Interestingly, confocal immunofluorescence imaging of a single tumor cell, as shown in Figure 5d, co-incubating gold salt and the shRNA1 similarly increased the number of RFP-LC3 positive dots (red), while decreased the number of LAMP2 positive spots (green). The number of p62 positive spots increased in shRNA1 and gold salt transfected cells, while the ratio of p62-LAMP2 pooled (merge) spots/p62 spots decreased compared to other cells (seen in Figure 5e). In addition, RFP-positive/p62 puncta were partly colocalized with LAMP2 in HepG2 cells co-incubated with gold salt and the shRNA1. Through bio-TEM and confocal imaging, the dynamics of autophagy flux and the expression changes of autophagy molecular markers in tumor cells are tracked to realize complex dynamic spatiotemporal analysis. Together, these results demonstrate that silencing of MALAT1 by Au–shRNA1 NCs inhibits autophagic flux.

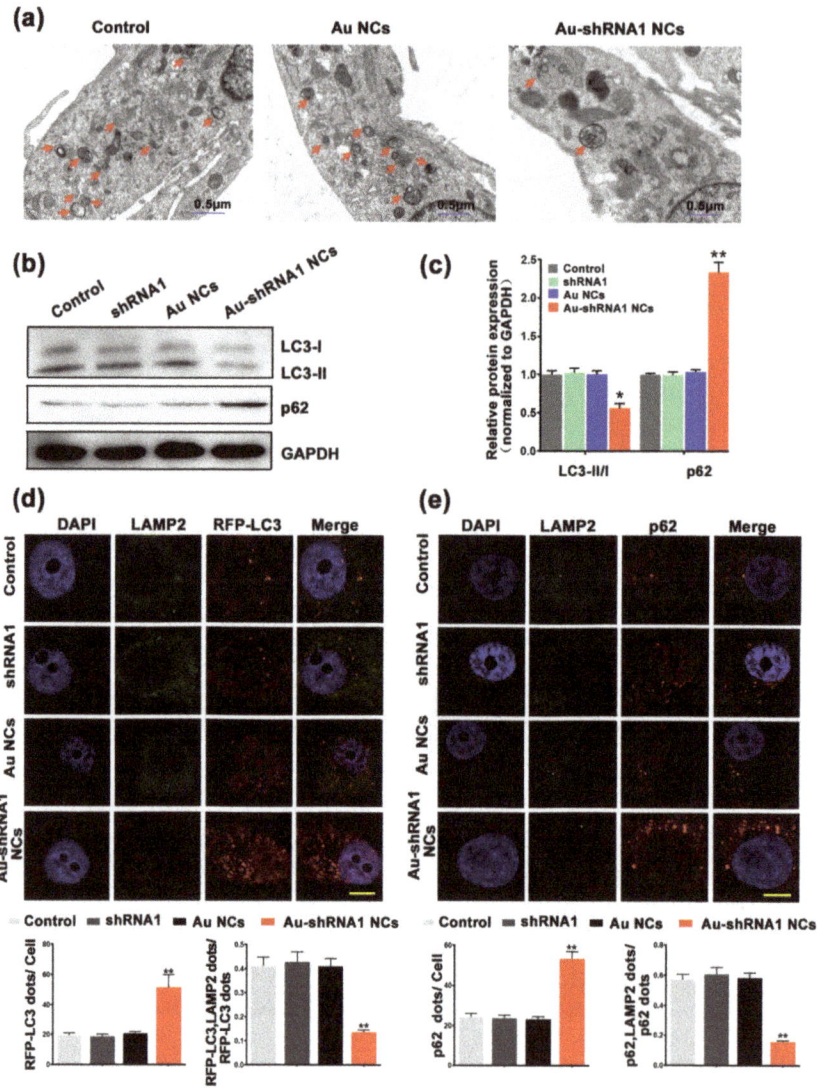

Figure 5. Silencing of MALAT1 by Au–shRNA1 NCs inhibits autophagic flux. (**a**) Bio-TEM images of HepG2 cells showing the accumulation of autophagosomes with or without gold salt treatment (bars = 0.5 μm). Red arrows indicate autophagosomes. (**b,c**) Western blot analysis was used to compare the expression levels of LC3 and p62 in the untreated control group, shRNA1, Au NC, and Au–shRNA1 NC groups. * $p < 0.05$, ** $p < 0.01$ (n = 3–5). (**d**) Representative images show RFP-LC3 and LAMP2 expression among different groups of HepG2 cells. Cells were first transfected with RFP-LC3 for 24 h, and then separately incubated with the shRNA1, gold salt, or the shRNA1 and gold salt together for 12 h. DAPI staining was applied to observe the cell nucleus. Scale bar: 5 μm. The figure shows the quantification of RFP-LC3 (red) dots. The bottom graph shows the combined point/RFP-LC3 ratio. ** $p < 0.01$ (n = 3–5). (**e**) Representative images of p62 and LAMP2 between different groups. The yellow dots in the merged image indicate the co-localization of LAMP2 and p62. Scale bar: 5 μm. The quantitative analysis of p62 (red) spots/cells and fusion spots/p62 in HepG2 cells is indicated (bottom). ** $p < 0.01$ (n = 3–5).

3.8. Au–shRNA1 NCs for Effective Bioimaging and Theranostics in an Orthotopic Tumor Model

Based on the cell experiments, we speculated that MALAT1-silenced cells had considerably lower pro-tumorigenic functions through reduced autophagy. To better understand and simulate the therapeutic effect of the synthesized Au–shRNA1 NCs, a xenograft tumor model was developed for further assessment. We inoculated xenograft tumors by injecting HepG2 cells and successfully established HCC tumor models (Figure S5a). We randomly divided the tumor model mice into four groups (i.e., the control, Au NC, shRNA1, and biosynthesized Au–shRNA1 NC groups), with four mice per group. We first explored whether self-assembled Au–shRNA1 NCs could be effectively delivered to tumors using real-time fluorescence imaging. According to the different experimental designs, the groups of mice were injected with different substances, and images were collected at 2–48 h (Figure 6a). The fluorescence intensity in the tumor tissue at different periods is shown in Figure 6b. The results show that self-assembled Au–shRNA1 NCs can achieve non-invasive fluorescence imaging of live animals and real-time detection of targeted tumors. The average intensity of the fluorescent signal increased with time and reaches a maximum in 24 h. In addition, the fluorescence signal of the Au–shRNA1 NC group was much higher than the Au NC group. Moreover, the resulting fluorescence was more intense in tumors, which further showed that the biosynthesized fluorescent Au–shRNA1 NCs were present in target tumors.

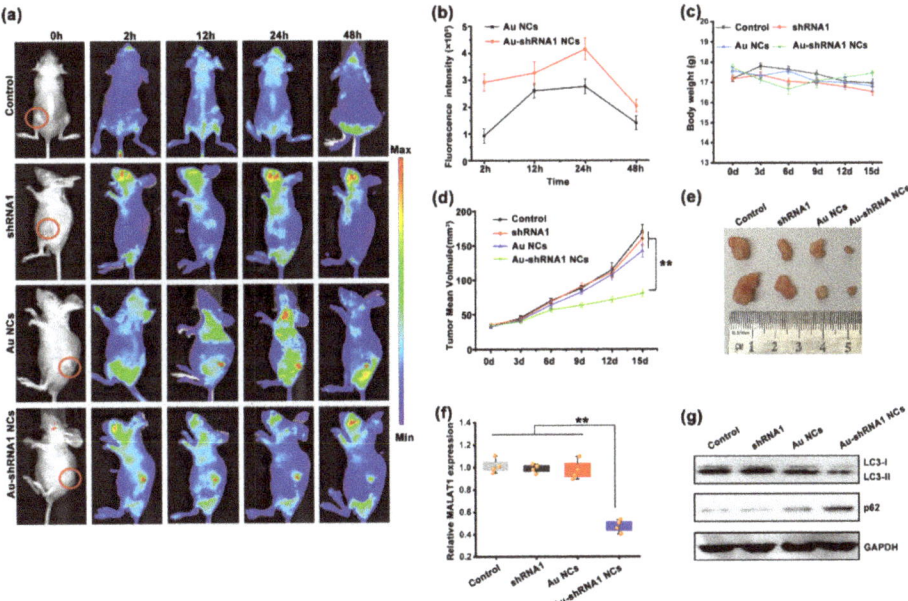

Figure 6. Silencing of MALAT1 by Au–shRNA1 NCs inhibits tumor proliferation in orthotopic tumor model via suppression of autophagic flux. (**a**) Dynamic biodistribution of normal saline (control), shRNA1, Au NCs, and Au–shRNA1 NCs in mice using fluorescent imaging at 0, 12, 24 and 48 h. (**b**) Fluorescence imaging of nude mice bearing HepG2 tumors at various time points after the injection of HAuCl$_4$ (black) or HAuCl$_4$ and shRNA1 (red) ($n = 4$). (**c**) Weights of each group of mice during the 15-day treatment. (**d**) HepG2 tumor growth in different time courses after treatment (ANOVA, ** $p < 0.01$). (**e**) Tumor images on day 15. (**f**) The expression of MALAT1 in tumor tissues of different treatment groups was detected by the qRT-PCR assay (** $p < 0.01$). (**g**) The expression of autophagy markers (LC3 and p62) in tumor tissues of different treatment groups was detected by western blot assay.

In addition to the above observations, we recorded the weights of the mice (Figure 6c). No remarkable differences were observed between the different groups during the treatment, suggesting few side effects. After five cycles of injection treatment, all nude mice were euthanized and xenograft tumors were collected for further analysis. Consistent with the results obtained in the in vitro cell experiment, the self-assembly biosynthesis Au–shRNA1 NC group showed enhanced inhibition of tumor growth (Figure 6d). The in situ self-assembled Au–shRNA1 NC treated group significantly reduced tumor volume (Figure 6e and Figure S5b,c). In addition, ex vivo imaging of mice treated with in situ synthesized Au NCs and Au–shRNA1 NCs showed that gold was mainly eliminated in vivo by the liver and kidneys (Figure S5d), which is consistent with previous reports [48,49].

Furthermore, we tested the mRNA levels of MALAT1 in different groups of tumor tissues to verify the ability of Au–shRNA1 NCs to silence MALAT1. As shown in Figure 6f, compared with that in the control groups treated with PBS, shRNA1 alone, or gold salt alone, the mRNA level of MALAT1 in the Au–shRNA1 NC group was significantly reduced. We then focused on the expression levels of p62 and LC3-II/I, which were measured in the aforementioned studies. The depletion of MALAT1 inhibited autophagy in tumor cells, and the western blot results showed that the LC3-II/I level in the Au–shRNA1 NC group was significantly reduced, while the p62 level was significantly increased compared with those in the control groups (Figure 6g). Moreover, to further evaluate the safety of the complex in vivo, we tested the biochemical parameters in the blood after the mice were killed (Figure S5e–i) and performed hematoxylin-eosin staining of the major organs (Figure S6). The results showed that the in situ biosynthetic Au–shRNA1 NCs had no obvious toxicity and did not cause damage to the liver or kidneys in mice.

4. Conclusions

shRNAs/siRNAs have great promise in disease treatment as potential drugs for silencing disease-related genes. However, due to the lack of effective and safe carriers, their usage is restricted. For cancer treatment, many major breakthroughs have been made in the past two decades, but there are still huge challenges. There is an urgent need to introduce safe and effective approaches for real-time bioimaging and monitoring of tumor development and treatments. At present, the application of bioimaging technology in clinical medical diagnosis has attracted much attention. The development of non-invasive in vivo imaging technology is an important prerequisite for its wide application in disease diagnosis and treatment. Furthermore, the participation of new fluorescent materials such as bio-self-assembly nanomaterials makes the application of imaging technology more accurate and biocompatible. Fluorescent nanomaterials have received increasing attention due to their unique physicochemical properties, and were used in medicine and other fields [50]. Nanocarriers as drug delivery systems are promising and have increased in popularity, especially for cancer treatment. Thus, with the help of bio-responsive molecular-level bioimaging technology, the development of a non-toxic, safe, and effective gold nanoparticle delivery system for shRNA/siRNA is critical to the clinical success of gene therapy.

Herein, we propose a novel method for shRNA delivery, imaging, and treatment of cancers using bio-responsive self-assembled fluorescent Au–shRNA NCs. It has significant advantages such as high targeting efficiency and high biocompatibility in precise tumor bioimaging and drug delivery systems. Its advantages in regulating cytotoxicity, cellular uptake, endosomal escape, and shRNA transfection efficiency may come from changing the balance between modules with different functions (e.g., electrostatic charge and pH) [51,52]. In situ self-assembled Au–shRNA NCs can protect shRNA from external effects, realize cellular uptake, and effective endosomal escape. In addition, the TEM and AFM images as well as the fluorescent characterization of these complexes, provide consistent evidence of in situ self-assembling Au–shRNA1 NCs. These observations support the formation of bio-responsive Au–shRNA1 NCs in vivo that form specifically in the unique cancer microenvironment [42,53,54].

Studies have demonstrated that MALAT1 is involved in the autophagy pathway and may be an inducer of autophagy [28,55,56]. More evidence shows that autophagy can help cancer cells overcome stress conditions, and tumor cells rely on autophagy as a survival strategy [57]. In this study, we used bio-self-assembled Au–shRNA1 NCs to silence MALAT1 and observed the resulting biological effects. In situ Au–shRNA1 NCs self-assembled in HepG2 HCC cells, and their various conformation states were further proven by TEM and AFM characterization. Furthermore, from a biological point of view, through a series of in vivo and in vitro related experiments and biological imaging, our observations demonstrated that the self-assembled fluorescence Au–shRNA1 NCs effectively bioimaged the diseased locations and silenced MALAT1, inhibiting the proliferation of HepG2 cells by suppressing autophagic flux (Figure 7).

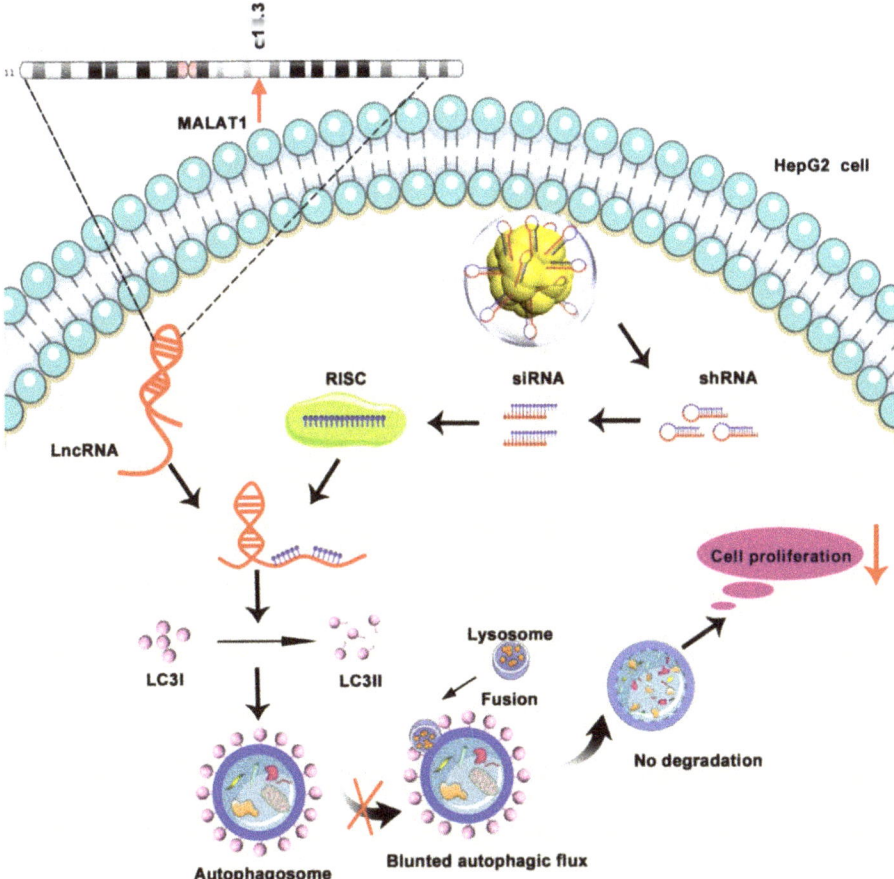

Figure 7. Schematic diagram of the potential mechanism by which Au–shRNA1 NCs effectively silence MALAT1 to inhibit the proliferation of HepG2 cells via the suppression of autophagy.

In summary, based on the observations above, our results demonstrate that the bio-responsive self-assembly Au–shRNA NCs could readily realize real-time cancer cell imaging and precise monitoring of tumor-targeting treatment from multi-scale levels, which can be further used to guide targeted cancer therapy. To the best of our knowledge, it is the first example to report a new shRNA self-assembled for a targeted nano-delivery system from the genetic level for non-invasive and effective cancer bioimaging and treatment.

MALAT1 is one of the star molecules of lncRNA and is upregulated in HCC; in this study, MALAT1-shRNA was first utilized to exploit the considerable efficiency of the in-situ bio-responsive self-assembly Au–shRNA NCs on silencing target gene MALAT1, which led to significant changes in autophagy. Meanwhile, when combined with bio-TEM and laser confocal imaging studies to track the dynamic changes of autophagic flux caused by the as-prepared Au–shRNA1NCs, it is exciting to realize high-resolution complex dynamic spatiotemporal analysis readily. This raises the possibility of facilitating accurate multi-scale bio-imaging from the molecular-level with target gene-recognition to cancer cell imaging and in vivo tumor tissue imaging for simultaneous precise targeted cancer therapy. In the future, we can further increase the sample size and more cell lines, combining them with the corresponding clinic samples. Thus, we believe that the ongoing cutting-edge studies will eventually provide a unique and promising theranostics strategy for cancer early diagnosis and precision treatment.

Supplementary Materials: The following are available online at https://www.mdpi.com/article/10.3390/bios11110425/s1, Figure S1: Elevated expression of MALAT1 identified in HCC. Figure S2: Analysis of the effect of different inhibitors on the uptake of Au–shRNA NCs by live HepG2 cells. Figure S3: Analysis of the tumor cell apoptosis rate in different groups (TUNEL staining). Figure S4: Representative laser confocal fluorescence images of L02 cells cultured with shRNA1 and gold salt. Figure S5: Au–shRNA NCs to achieve biological effects for tumor mice imaging and theranostics. Figure S6: Tissue sections of major dissected organs from different treatment groups were stained with H&E. Table S1: Correlations between MALAT1 expression and clinicopathological characteristics in 30 HCC tissues. Table S2: Sequences of shRNA and lncRNA primers. Table S3: The antibodies employed for western blot analysis.

Author Contributions: Conceptualization, W.C., Y.W. and X.W.; Investigation, W.C. and L.Y.; Supervision, Y.W. and X.W.; Validation, H.J.; Writing—original draft, W.C. and L.Y.; Writing—review & editing, Y.W. and X.W. All authors have read and agreed to the published version of the manuscript.

Funding: This work was supported by the National Natural Science Foundation of China (82061148012, 82027806, 91753106), the National Key Research and Development Program of China (2017YFA0205300), and the Primary Research & Development Plan of Jiangsu Province (BE2019716). This work was also supported by the ISF-NSFC Joint Research Program (grant no. 3258/20) to Y.W.

Institutional Review Board Statement: Not applicable.

Informed Consent Statement: Not applicable.

Data Availability Statement: Not applicable.

Acknowledgments: We sincerely thank the patients as well as the medical staff in the First Affiliated Hospital, Shihezi University School of Medicine involved in collecting specimens.

Conflicts of Interest: The authors declare no conflict of interest.

References

1. Esteller, M. Non-coding RNAs in human disease. *Nat. Rev. Genet.* **2011**, *12*, 861–874. [CrossRef]
2. Quinn, J.J.; Chang, H.Y. Unique features of long non-coding RNA biogenesis and function. *Nat. Rev. Genet.* **2015**, *17*, 47–62. [CrossRef]
3. Geisler, S.; Coller, J. RNA in unexpected places: Long non-coding RNA functions in diverse cellular contexts. *Nat. Rev. Mol. Cell Biol.* **2013**, *14*, 699–712. [CrossRef] [PubMed]
4. E Kornienko, A.; Guenzl, P.M.; Barlow, D.P.; Pauler, F.M. Gene regulation by the act of long non-coding RNA transcription. *BMC Biol.* **2013**, *11*, 59. [CrossRef]
5. Wong, C.-M.; Tsang, F.H.-C.; Ng, I.O.-L. Non-coding RNAs in hepatocellular carcinoma: Molecular functions and pathological implications. *Nat. Rev. Gastroenterol. Hepatol.* **2018**, *15*, 137–151. [CrossRef]
6. Cesana, M.; Cacchiarelli, D.; Legnini, I.; Santini, T.; Sthandier, O.; Chinappi, M.; Tramontano, A.; Bozzoni, I. A long noncoding RNA controls muscle differentiation by functioning as a competing endogenous RNA. *Cell* **2011**, *147*, 358–369. [CrossRef] [PubMed]
7. Fang, Y.; Fullwood, M.J. Roles, Functions, and Mechanisms of Long Non-coding RNAs in Cancer. *Genom. Proteom. Bioinform.* **2016**, *14*, 42–54. [CrossRef]

8. Mercer, T.; Dinger, M.; Mattick, J. Long non-coding RNAs: Insights into functions. *Nat. Rev. Genet.* **2009**, *10*, 155–159. [CrossRef] [PubMed]
9. Wang, K.C.; Chang, H.Y. Molecular Mechanisms of Long Noncoding RNAs. *Mol. Cell* **2011**, *43*, 904–914. [CrossRef] [PubMed]
10. Jiang, M.-C.; Ni, J.-J.; Cui, W.-Y.; Wang, B.-Y.; Zhuo, W. Emerging roles of lncRNA in cancer and therapeutic opportunities. *Am. J. Cancer Res.* **2019**, *9*, 1354–1366. [PubMed]
11. Yiren, H.; Yingcong, Y.; Sunwu, Y.; Keqin, L.; XiaoChun, T.; Senrui, C.; Ende, C.; Xizhou, L.; Yanfan, C. Long noncoding RNA MALAT1 regulates autophagy associated chemoresistance via miR-23b-3p sequestration in gastric cancer. *Mol. Cancer* **2017**, *16*, 174. [CrossRef] [PubMed]
12. Song, W.; Zhang, R.J.; Zou, S.B. Long noncoding RNA MALAT1 as a potential novel biomarker in digestive system cancers: A meta-analysis. *Minerva Med.* **2016**, *107*, 245–250. [PubMed]
13. Shi, X.S.; Li, J.; Yang, R.H.; Zhao, G.R.; Zhou, H.P.; Zeng, W.X.; Zhou, M. Correlation of increased MALAT1 expression with pathological fea-tures and prognosis in cancer patients: A meta-analysis. *Genet. Mol. Res.* **2015**, *14*, 18808–18819. [CrossRef] [PubMed]
14. Wang, J.; Xu, A.; Zhang, J.; He, X.; Pan, Y.; Cheng, G.; Qin, C.; Hua, L.; Wang, Z. Prognostic significance of long non-coding RNA MALAT-1 in various human carcinomas: A meta-analysis. *Genet. Mol. Res.* **2016**, *15*, gmr-15017433. [CrossRef]
15. Fujimoto, A.; Furuta, M.; Totoki, Y.; Tsunoda, T.; Kato, M.; Shiraishi, Y.; Tanaka, H.; Taniguchi, H.; Kawakami, Y.; Ueno, M.; et al. Whole-genome mutational landscape and characterization of noncoding and structural mutations in liver cancer. *Nat. Genet.* **2016**, *48*, 500–509. [CrossRef]
16. Kim, B.; Park, J.; Sailor, M.J. Rekindling RNAi Therapy: Materials Design Requirements for In Vivo siRNA Delivery. *Adv. Mater.* **2019**, *31*, e1903637. [CrossRef] [PubMed]
17. Alterman, J.F.; Godinho, B.M.D.C.; Hassler, M.R.; Ferguson, C.M.; Echeverria, D.; Sapp, E.; Haraszti, R.A.; Coles, A.H.; Conroy, F.; Miller, R.; et al. A divalent siRNA chemical scaffold for potent and sustained modulation of gene expression throughout the central nervous system. *Nat. Biotechnol.* **2019**, *37*, 884–894. [CrossRef] [PubMed]
18. Lambeth, L.S.; Smith, C.A. Short Hairpin RNA-Mediated Gene Silencing. *Methods Mol. Biol.* **2012**, *942*, 205–232. [CrossRef]
19. Patra, J.K.; Das, G.; Fraceto, L.F.; Campos, E.V.R.; Rodriguez-Torres, M.D.P.; Acosta-Torres, L.S.; Diaz-Torres, L.A.; Grillo, R.; Swamy, M.K.; Sharma, S.; et al. Nano based drug delivery systems: Recent developments and future prospects. *J. Nanobiotechnol.* **2018**, *16*, 71. [CrossRef] [PubMed]
20. Sharma, A.; Jha, N.K.; Dahiya, K.; Singh, V.K.; Chaurasiya, K.; Jha, A.N.; Jha, S.K.; Mishra, P.C.; Dholpuria, S.; Astya, R.; et al. Nanoparticulate RNA delivery systems in cancer. *Cancer Rep.* **2020**, *3*, e1271. [CrossRef]
21. Liu, C.-J.; Chen, P.-J. Elimination of Hepatitis B in Highly Endemic Settings: Lessons Learned in Taiwan and Challenges Ahead. *Viruses* **2020**, *12*, 815. [CrossRef] [PubMed]
22. Wu, Q.; Qin, S.-K. Features and treatment options of Chinese hepatocellular carcinoma. *Chin. Clin. Oncol.* **2013**, *2*, 38. [CrossRef] [PubMed]
23. Fu, S.; Wang, Y.; Li, H.; Chen, L.; Liu, Q. Regulatory Networks of LncRNA MALAT-1 in Cancer. *Cancer Manag. Res.* **2020**, *12*, 10181–10198. [CrossRef]
24. Guerrieri, F. Long non-coding RNAs era in liver cancer. *World J. Hepatol.* **2015**, *7*, 1971–1973. [CrossRef] [PubMed]
25. LaiZhe, M.-C.; Yang, Z.; Zhou, L.; Zhu, Q.-Q.; Xie, H.-Y.; Zhang, F.; Wu, L.-M.; Chen, L.-M.; Zheng, S.-S. Long non-coding RNA MALAT-1 overexpression predicts tumor recurrence of hepatocellular carcinoma after liver transplantation. *Med. Oncol.* **2011**, *29*, 1810–1816. [CrossRef]
26. Galluzzi, L.; Pietrocola, F.; Levine, B.; Kroemer, G. Metabolic Control of Autophagy. *Cell* **2014**, *159*, 1263–1276. [CrossRef]
27. Wang, K.; Liu, C.-Y.; Zhou, L.-Y.; Wang, J.; Wang, M.; Zhao, B.; Zhao, W.-K.; Jian-Xun, W.; Yan-Fang, Z.; Zhang, X.-J.; et al. APF lncRNA regulates autophagy and myocardial infarction by targeting miR-188-3p. *Nat. Commun.* **2015**, *6*, 6779. [CrossRef] [PubMed]
28. Li, L.; Chen, H.; Gao, Y.; Wang, Y.-W.; Zhang, G.-Q.; Pan, S.-H.; Ji, L.; Kong, R.; Wang, G.; Jia, Y.-H.; et al. Long Noncoding RNA MALAT1 Promotes Aggressive Pancreatic Cancer Proliferation and Metastasis via the Stimulation of Autophagy. *Mol. Cancer Ther.* **2016**, *15*, 2232–2243. [CrossRef] [PubMed]
29. Yip, K.M.; Fischer, N.; Paknia, E.; Chari, A.; Stark, H. Atomic-resolution protein structure determination by cryo-EM. *Nature* **2020**, *587*, 157–161. [CrossRef] [PubMed]
30. Prabhakar, N.; Peurla, M.; Shenderova, O.; Rosenholm, J.M. Fluorescent and Electron-Dense Green Color Emitting Nanodiamonds for Single-Cell Correlative Microscopy. *Molecules* **2020**, *25*, 5897. [CrossRef]
31. Cai, W.; Feng, H.; Yin, L.; Wang, M.; Jiang, X.; Qin, Z.; Liu, W.; Li, C.; Jiang, H.; Weizmann, Y.; et al. Bio responsive self-assembly of Au-miRNAs for targeted cancer theranostics. *EBioMedicine* **2020**, *54*, 102740. [CrossRef]
32. Wang, M.; Chen, Y.; Cai, W.; Feng, H.; Du, T.; Liu, W.; Jiang, H.; Pasquarelli, A.; Weizmann, Y.; Wang, X. In situ self-assembling Au-DNA com-plexes for targeted cancer bioimaging and inhibition. *Proc. Natl. Acad. Sci. USA* **2020**, *117*, 308–316. [CrossRef] [PubMed]
33. Rhodes, D.R.; Kalyana-Sundaram, S.; Mahavisno, V.; Varambally, R.; Yu, J.; Briggs, B.B.; Barrette, T.R.; Anstet, M.J.; Kincead-Beal, C.; Kulkarni, P.; et al. Oncomine 3.0: Genes, pathways, and networks in a collection of 18,000 cancer gene expres-sion profiles. *Neoplasia* **2007**, *9*, 166–180. [CrossRef] [PubMed]

34. Xie, Z.-C.; Dang, Y.-W.; Wei, D.-M.; Chen, P.; Tang, R.-X.; Huang, Q.; Liu, J.-H.; Luo, D.-Z. Clinical significance and prospective molecular mechanism of MALAT1 in pancreatic cancer exploration: A comprehensive study based on the GeneChip, GEO, Oncomine, and TCGA databases. *OncoTargets Ther.* **2017**, *10*, 3991–4005. [CrossRef]
35. Chen, X.; Cheung, S.T.; So, S.; Fan, S.T.; Barry, C.; Higgins, J.; Lai, K.-M.; Ji, J.; Dudoit, S.; Ng, I.O.-L.; et al. Gene Expression Patterns in Human Liver Cancers. *Mol. Biol. Cell* **2002**, *13*, 1929–1939. [CrossRef] [PubMed]
36. Wurmbach, E.; Chen, Y.-B.; Khitrov, G.; Zhang, W.; Roayaie, S.; Schwartz, M.; Fiel, I.; Thung, S.; Mazzaferro, V.M.; Bruix, J.; et al. Genome-wide molecular profiles of HCV-induced dysplasia and hepatocellular carcinoma. *Hepatology* **2007**, *45*, 938–947. [CrossRef] [PubMed]
37. Gao, Y.; Shang, S.; Guo, S.; Li, X.; Zhou, H.; Liu, H.; Sun, Y.; Wang, J.; Wang, P.; Zhi, H.; et al. Lnc2Cancer 3.0: An updated re-source for experimentally supported lncRNA/circRNA cancer associations and web tools based on RNA-seq and scRNA-seq data. *Nucleic Acids Res.* **2021**, *49*, D1251–D1258. [CrossRef]
38. Dou, J.; Gu, N. Emerging strategies for the identification and targeting of cancer stem cells. *Tumor Biol.* **2010**, *31*, 243–253. [CrossRef]
39. Rehman, F.U.; Du, T.; Shaikh, S.; Jiang, X.; Chen, Y.; Li, X.; Yi, H.; Hui, J.; Chen, B.; Selke, M.; et al. Nano in nano: Biosynthesized gold and iron nanoclusters cargo neoplastic exosomes for cancer status biomarking. *Nanomed. Nanotechnol. Biol. Med.* **2018**, *14*, 2619–2631. [CrossRef]
40. Wang, J.; Zhang, G.; Li, Q.; Jiang, H.; Liu, C.; Amatore, C.; Wang, X. In vivo self-bio-imaging of tumors through in situ biosynthesized fluo-rescent gold nanoclusters. *Sci. Rep.* **2013**, *3*, 1157. [CrossRef]
41. Chang, H.-C.; Wang, X.; Shiu, K.-K.; Zhu, Y.; Wang, J.; Li, Q.; Chen, B.; Jiang, H. Layer-by-layer assembly of graphene, Au and poly(toluidine blue O) films sensor for evaluation of oxidative stress of tumor cells elicited by hydrogen peroxide. *Biosens. Bioelectron.* **2013**, *41*, 789–794. [CrossRef]
42. Szatrowski, T.P.; Nathan, C.F. Production of large amounts of hydrogen peroxide by human tumor cells. *Cancer Res.* **1991**, *51*, 794–798.
43. Sajid, M.I.; Moazzam, M.; Kato, S.; Cho, K.Y.; Tiwari, R.K. Overcoming Barriers for siRNA Therapeutics: From Bench to Bedside. *Pharmaceuticals* **2020**, *13*, 294. [CrossRef] [PubMed]
44. Pei, D.; Buyanova, M. Overcoming Endosomal Entrapment in Drug Delivery. *Bioconjugate Chem.* **2018**, *30*, 273–283. [CrossRef] [PubMed]
45. Si, Y.; Yang, Z.; Ge, Q.; Yu, L.; Yao, M.; Sun, X.; Ren, Z.; Ding, C. Long non-coding RNA Malat1 activated autophagy, hence promoting cell pro-liferation and inhibiting apoptosis by sponging miR-101 in colorectal cancer. *Cell Mol. Biol. Lett.* **2019**, *24*, 50. [CrossRef] [PubMed]
46. Galluzzi, L.; Green, D.R. Autophagy-Independent Functions of the Autophagy Machinery. *Cell* **2019**, *177*, 1682–1699. [CrossRef]
47. Johansen, T.; Lamark, T. Selective autophagy mediated by autophagic adapter proteins. *Autophagy* **2011**, *7*, 279–296. [CrossRef]
48. Sancey, L.; Kotb, S.; Truillet, C.; Appaix, F.; Marais, A.; Thomas, E.; van der Sanden, B.; Klein, J.-P.; Laurent, B.; Cottier, M.; et al. Long-Term in Vivo Clearance of Gadolinium-Based AGuIX Nanoparticles and Their Biocompatibility after Systemic Injection. *ACS Nano* **2015**, *9*, 2477–2488. [CrossRef]
49. Yu, M.; Xu, J.; Zheng, J. Renal Clearable Luminescent Gold Nanoparticles: From the Bench to the Clinic. *Angew. Chem. Int. Ed.* **2018**, *58*, 4112–4128. [CrossRef]
50. Kapara, A.; Brunton, V.; Graham, D.; Faulds, K. Investigation of cellular uptake mechanism of functionalised gold nanoparticles into breast cancer using SERS. *Chem. Sci.* **2020**, *11*, 5819–5829. [CrossRef] [PubMed]
51. Nelson, C.E.; Kintzing, J.R.; Hanna, A.; Shannon, J.M.; Gupta, M.K.; Duvall, C.L. Balancing Cationic and Hydrophobic Content of PEGylated siRNA Polyplexes Enhances Endosome Escape, Stability, Blood Circulation Time, and Bioactivity in Vivo. *ACS Nano* **2013**, *7*, 8870–8880. [CrossRef] [PubMed]
52. Zheng, M.; Librizzi, D.; Kılıç, A.; Liu, Y.; Renz, H.; Merkel, O.M.; Kissel, T. Enhancing in vivo circulation and siRNA delivery with biodegradable polyethylenimine-graft-polycaprolactone-block-poly(ethylene glycol) copolymers. *Biomaterials* **2012**, *33*, 6551–6558. [CrossRef] [PubMed]
53. Bao, B.; Azmi, A.; Li, Y.; Ahmad, A.; Ali, S.; Banerjee, S.; Kong, D.; Sarkar, F. Targeting CSCs in Tumor Microenvironment: The Potential Role of ROS-Associated miRNAs in Tumor Aggressiveness. *Curr. Stem Cell Res. Ther.* **2013**, *9*, 22–35. [CrossRef] [PubMed]
54. Feng, Q.; Li, Y.; Yang, X.; Zhang, W.; Hao, Y.; Zhang, H.; Hou, L.; Zhang, Z. Hypoxia-specific therapeutic agents delivery nanotheranostics: A sequential strategy for ultrasound mediated on-demand tritherapies and imaging of cancer. *J. Control. Release* **2018**, *275*, 192–200. [CrossRef]
55. Li, Z.; Li, J.; Tang, N. Long noncoding RNA Malat1 is a potent autophagy inducer protecting brain microvascular endothelial cells against oxygen-glucose deprivation/reoxygenation-induced injury by sponging miR-26b and upregulating ULK2 expression. *Neuroscience* **2017**, *354*, 1–10. [CrossRef] [PubMed]
56. Yuan, P.; Cao, W.; Zang, Q.; Li, G.; Guo, X.; Fan, J. The HIF-2α-MALAT1-miR-216b axis regulates multi-drug resistance of hepatocellular carcinoma cells via modulating autophagy. *Biochem. Biophys. Res. Commun.* **2016**, *478*, 1067–1073. [CrossRef]
57. Huang, Z.; Zhou, L.; Chen, Z.; Nice, E.C.; Huang, C. Stress management by autophagy: Implications for chemoresistance. *Int. J. Cancer* **2016**, *139*, 23–32. [CrossRef] [PubMed]

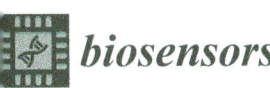

Article

Aptamer Embedded Arch-Cruciform DNA Assemblies on 2-D VS$_2$ Scaffolds for Sensitive Detection of Breast Cancer Cells

Jinfeng Quan [1,†], Yihan Wang [1,†], Jialei Zhang [1], Kejing Huang [2], Xuemei Wang [1,*] and Hui Jiang [1,*]

1 State Key Laboratory of Bioelectronics, National Demonstration Center for Experimental Biomedical Engineering Education, School of Biological Science and Medical Engineering, Southeast University, Nanjing 210096, China; jfquan0224@163.com (J.Q.); yihanwangxynu@163.com (Y.W.); 220181811@seu.edu.cn (J.Z.)
2 School of Chemistry and Chemical Engineering, Guangxi University for Nationalities, Nanning 530008, China; kejinghuang@163.com
* Correspondence: xuewang@seu.edu.cn (X.W.); sungi@seu.edu.cn (H.J.)
† These authors are contributed equally to this work.

Abstract: Arch-cruciform DNA are self-assembled on AuNPs/VS$_2$ scaffold as a highly sensitive and selective electrochemical biosensor for michigan cancer foundation-7 (MCF-7) breast cancer cells. In the construction, arch DNA is formed using two single-strand DNA sequences embedded with the aptamer for MCF-7 cells. In the absence of MCF-7 cells, a cruciform DNA labeled with three terminal biotin is bound to the top of arch DNA, which further combines with streptavidin-labeled horseradish peroxidase (HRP) to catalyze the hydroquinone-H$_2$O$_2$ reaction on the electrode surface. The presence of MCF-7 cells can release the cruciform DNA and reduce the amount of immobilized HRP, thus effectively inhibiting enzyme-mediated electrocatalysis. The electrochemical response of the sensor is negatively correlated with the concentration of MCF-7 cells, with a linear range of 10~1 × 10^5 cells/mL, and a limit of detection as low as 5 cells/mL (S/N = 3). Through two-dimensional materials and enzyme-based dual signal amplification, this biosensor may pave new ways for the highly sensitive detection of tumor cells in real samples.

Keywords: MCF-7 cells; electrochemistry; 2-D materials; signal amplification; DNA assembly

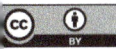

1. Introduction

Breast cancer is the fifth leading cause of death among all cancers, and it is also the most common non-skin cancer in women [1,2]. The breast cancer cell line can be classified based on the status of three important receptors, including estrogen receptor (ER), progesterone receptor (PR), and human epithelial receptor-2 (HER2) [3]. MCF-7 (ER+PR+HER2-), a typical breast cancer cell line, accounts for more than two-thirds of the cell lines used in related studies, along with T47-D and MDA-MB-231 cells, which have been widely used for breast cancer modelling. It is noteworthy that breast cancer cells can endanger the lives of patients through proliferation and metastasis over a short time. Early diagnosis and treatment can be helpful to better understand the patients' condition, and make appropriate treatment plan according to the degree of disease, which is very important to improve the survival rate of breast cancer [4–6].

At present, there are several common breast cancer screening methods, including computed tomography (CT) [7,8], magnetic resonance imaging (MRI) [9,10], positron emission computed tomography (PET) [11,12] and flow cytometry [13]. However, these techniques are usually expensive and time-consuming, and can lead to false-positive or negative results due to limited resolution [14]. Therefore, it is necessary to develop alternative molecular biological methods with high sensitivity, high accuracy and low cost for breast cancer diagnosis. There are numerous methods to detect MCF-7, including electrochemistry [15], electrochemiluminescence [16], colorimetry [17] and photoelectrochemical methods [18].

Aptamers, which are single-stranded DNA or RNA analogues to antibodies [19], have been attracting a lot of interest due to their advantages over traditional recognition molecules. As the recognition probe for cancer cells, aptamers can specifically bind and recognize proteins on the surface of cancer cells [4,20,21]. Based on aptamers, highly sensitive and selective biosensors can be constructed for the detection of MCF-7 cancer cells.

For this purpose, a careful choice needs to be made with regard to biosensing elements with multiple amplification capacity. The first issue is to seek an efficient scaffold to support the physical or biochemical amplification. Recently, two-dimensional (2D) matrices have received tremendous interest [22–24]. Among them, vanadium disulfide (VS_2) is the most common vanadium-based transition metal dichalcogenide [25]. VS_2 nanosheets have excellent conductivity and have been well used in high-performance rechargeable metal ion batteries with abundant metal ion storage sites and low ion diffusion barriers [26–28], photoelectrochemical water splitting and solar cells [29,30]. More importantly, VS_2 has a high specific surface area and superior mechanical properties, which is conducive to the construction of an effective biosensor platform. For example, Tian et al. [31] constructed an electrochemical aptasensor for kanamycin based on VS_2/AuNPs nanocomposites and $CoFe_2O_4$ nanoenzyme as signal amplifiers. The recognition of kanamycin by aptamers results in the decrease in nanoenzyme accumulation and the increase in electrochemical signals by methylene blue. Actually, it may be more rational to design aptasensors depending on both VS_2 nanosheets and the self-assembled complementary DNA sequences.

Hence, this work aims to construct a highly sensitive human breast MCF-7 cancer cell sensing platform with synergistic amplification by both VS_2 nanocomposites and aptamer-binding enzyme (Scheme 1). Firstly, AuNPs are electrodeposited on the surfaces of VS_2 nanosheets to fabricate an ideal electrochemical scaffold. Then, the arch DNA aptamer that specifically binds to MCF-7 cells is self-assembled on this scaffold through the well-known gold-thiolate interaction. In the absence of MCF-7 cells, the immobilized arch DNA is hybridized with biotin-labeled cruciform DNA and further linked with biotinylated horseradish peroxidase (HRP), which may catalyze the reaction of hydrogen peroxide (H_2O_2) and hydroquinone (HQ) to produce electrochemical signals. Target MCF-7 cells may compete with the cruciform DNA for the binding site of the arch DNA aptamer, and cause the release of the cruciform DNA, which further inhibits the immobilization of HRP on the electrode, thus reducing the electrochemical response. Based on this principle, the concentration of MCF-7 cells can be detected by the electrochemical signals. This biosensor may pave new ways for the highly sensitive detection of tumor cells in real samples.

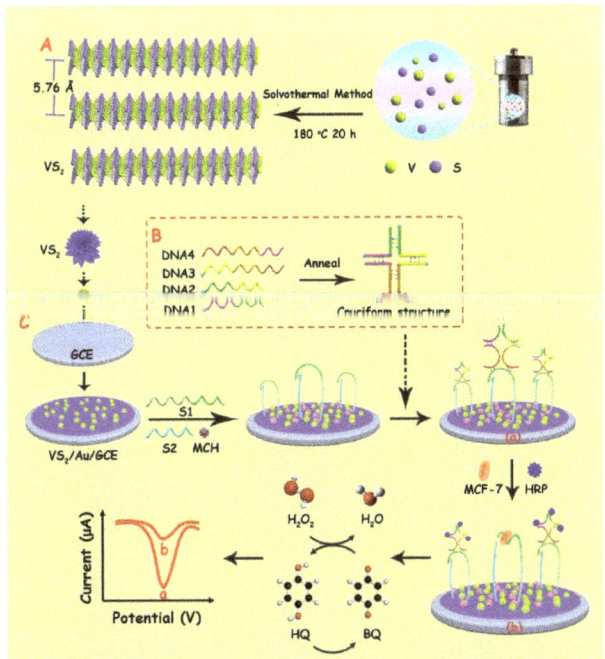

Scheme 1. Illustration of highly sensitive breast cancer cell sensor based on VS$_2$.

2. Materials and Methods

2.1. Reagents and Instruments

Sodium orthovanadate (Na$_3$VO$_4$·12H$_2$O), H$_2$O$_2$, 6-mercaptohexanol (MCH), horseradish peroxidase (HRP), and anhydrous ethanol were purchased from Sinopharm Chemical Reagent Co., Ltd. (Shanghai, China). Thioacetamide (CH$_3$CSNH$_2$), HQ, HAuCl$_4$·4H$_2$O, tris-(2-carboxyethyl) phosphine hydrochloride (TCEP) were purchased from Aladdin Co., Ltd. (Shanghai, China). All DNA strands used were purchased from Sangon Biotechnology Co., Ltd. (Shanghai, China), and the base sequences are listed in Table S1 (Supplementary Materials).

The details of instruments are listed in Table S2. The electrochemical experimental conditions and parameters are shown in Table S3.

2.2. Preparation of VS$_2$ Nanosheets

VS$_2$ nanosheets were prepared by the hydrothermal method. In a typical reaction, the precursors of sodium orthovanadate (2.36 g) and thioacetamide (2.79 g) were slowly dissolved in 60 mL of distilled water, and continuously stirred for 30 min to obtain a uniform solution. The solution was transferred to a 100 mL autoclave and kept at 180 °C for 20 h. After the reaction system was cooled to room temperature, the collected black precipitates were washed and centrifuged 3 times and dried at 60 °C for 12 h.

2.3. Preparation of Cruciform DNA

The cruciform DNA probe was assembled by four single strands of DNA, namely, DNA1, DNA2, DNA3 and DNA4. Firstly, the four single chains were mixed in the same molar ratio, and the final concentration of cruciform DNA was 1 μmol/L. Then, the mixture was heated to 95 °C for 10 min, and gradually cooled to 4 °C to obtain cruciform DNA probe by annealing steps (part B, Scheme 1). The successful preparation of cruciform DNA was verified by gel electrophoresis (Figure S2B). The cytotoxic assays also demonstrate the excellent biosafety of cruciform DNA (Figure S2A).

2.4. Cytotoxicity Test of Arch and Cruciform DNA

MCF-7 cells were seeded in 96-well plates at 1×10^4/well. After 24 h, the cells completely adhered to the well and the medium was removed. After 24 h incubation with different concentrations of arch DNA and cruciform DNA, 10 μL CCK-8 solution was added in each well and incubated at 37 °C for 2 h in dark. The optical density of each well at 450 nm was measured by microplate, and the cell survival rate was calculated [32].

2.5. Preparation of Biosensor

Firstly, glassy carbon electrode (GCE) was pretreated with aluminum oxide powder, cleaned and dried. VS_2 suspension (1 mg/mL) was dripped on the electrode surface and dried in air to obtain VS_2/GCE. Then, VS_2/GCE was immersed in a mixed solution containing 0.1% $HAuCl_4$ and 0.1 mol/L KCl, and AuNPs were electrodeposited by the amperometric I-t method with deposition voltage of −0.2 V and deposition time of 25 s [33]. AuNPs were in situ synthesized on the electrode surface to form AuNPs/VS_2/GCE. The mixed aptamer solution was obtained by dissolving 1 μmol/L aptamer S1 and 1 μmol/L aptamer S2 in Tris-HCl buffer of pH 7.0 (containing 50 mmol/L NaCl, 10 mmol/L $MgCl_2$, and 10 mmol/L TCEP). An amount of 10 μL of the above mixed solution was coated on AuNPs/VS_2/GCE and incubated at room temperature for 12 h. Both DNA strands were immobilized on the electrode by Au-S bond and electrostatic interaction. Note that S1 and S2 have complementary tail sequences to form arched DNA. After washing with distilled water, MCH (5 μL, 1 mmol/L) was incubated on the electrode surface for 30 min to block the active sites and inhibit the non-specific adsorption. An amount of 8 μL cruciform DNA probe was then modified on the electrode surface by incubation at 37 °C for 80 min, in virtue of the hybridization of cruciform DNA to the top of arch DNA. At each modification step, the electrode was washed with Tris-HCl buffer (pH = 7.4) to remove the unbound molecules.

For cellular measurements, different concentrations of cell suspension of 8 μL were incubated at room temperature for 100 min, and the aptamer S1 was used to capture the cells. Subsequently, 8 μL HRP (10 μg/mL) labeled with streptavidin was immobilized on the electrode surface at 37 °C for 30 min and bound to the cruciform DNA surface by biotin–streptavidin interaction. For DPV tests, the electrodes were placed in 10 mL 0.1 mol/L PBS (pH 5.0) containing 1.8 mmol/L H_2O_2 and 2 mmol/L HQ, respectively.

3. Results and Discussion

3.1. Characterization of VS_2

The morphology of VS_2 is characterized in Figure 1. The SEM images show that a large number of 2D VS_2 nanosheets are stacked and interwoven to form a flower-like structure (Figure 1A,B). These nanosheets are uniform in thickness (~30 nm) and the diameter ranges from 0.5 to 1 μm. The TEM image in Figure 1C show that single flower-like VS_2 is composed of loosely arranged nanosheets, which are connected by the center to form three-dimensional layers. The thin layer extends outwards and provides an excellent electron transfer interface. Figure 1D shows a high-resolution transmission electron microscope (HR-TEM) image inside a nanoplate, showing that the interlayer spacing is about 0.576 and 0.253 nm, corresponding to the (001) and (011) crystal plane of VS_2 [34], respectively.

The distribution of elemental components in VS_2 was studied by energy-dispersive X-ray spectroscopy (EDS) (Figure 2A). The results show the presence of V, S, C, and O on the surface of substrate. The atomic number ratio of V to S is about 1:1.95, which is very close to the theoretical atomic number ratio of 1:2 of VS_2, indicating a high purity. The XRD results (Figure 2B) show that the diffraction peaks of VS_2 nanosheets are located at 15.41°, 36.12°, 45.46°, 57.15°, 69.23° and 75.25°, which can be attributed to the corresponding diffraction crystal planes of (001), (011), (012), (110), (201) and (202), respectively, for the hexagonal phase of 2H-VS_2 (JPCDS No. 89-1640). Moreover, the sharp (011) diffraction peak proves that VS_2 has good crystallinity and layered structure [27]. In Raman spectroscopy, the characteristic peaks of VS_2 are 138.71 cm^{-1}, 192.25 cm^{-1}, 282.67 cm^{-1}, 404.24 cm^{-1},

686.58 cm^{-1} and 991.42 cm^{-1} in the range of 100~1100 cm^{-1} (Figure 2C). Typically, the peaks at 138.71 cm^{-1} and 192.25 cm^{-1} can be attributed to the vibration dispersion of VS$_2$. The characteristic peak at 282.67 cm^{-1} corresponds to the plane (E_{1g}) vibration mode in VS$_2$, which is the opposite vibration of two S atoms relative to V atoms in the plane; the peak at 404.24 cm^{-1} corresponds to the out of plane (A_{1g}) vibration mode of the S atom along the c axis [34]. The small half peak width and high intensity of these peaks also indicate that the VS$_2$ samples are in a highly crystalline state. The XPS (Figure 2D) also shows the V, S, C and O elements in samples, which is consistent with the EDS results. The two binding energy peaks of V 2p spectrum (Figure 2E) appear at 524.3 eV and 516.7 eV, which could correspond to the molecular orbits of V 2p$_{1/2}$ and V 2p$_{3/2}$, indicating that V exists at +4 valence in VS$_2$. The S 2p$_{3/2}$ and S 2p$_{1/2}$ peaks are located at 161.4 and 161.21 eV, respectively (Figure 2F), proving that the presence of −2 valence [30].

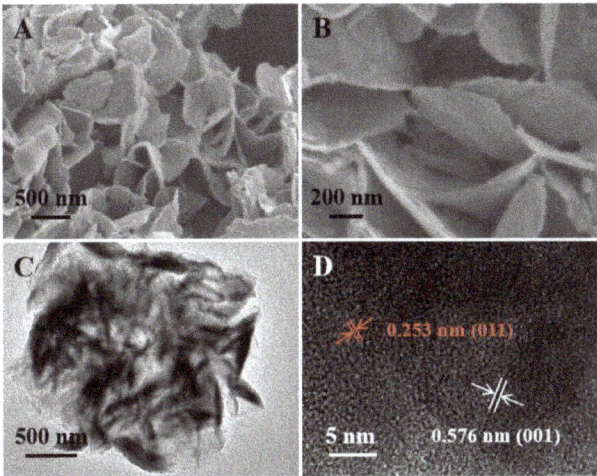

Figure 1. Morphological characterization of VS$_2$ nanosheets: (**A,B**) SEM images; (**C**)TEM image; (**D**) HR-TEM image.

3.2. Electrochemical Characterization

To fabricate the biosensor, we used a dual amplification strategy on the basis of AuNPs/VS$_2$ nanocomposites and enzyme, using aptamers with highly addressable and strong affinity, selectivity and stability. Considering that 2D and 3D DNA structures have stronger selective binding affinity and better stability compared to other common nucleic acid structures, an arch-cruciform-shaped DNA is introduced, which can combine with more enzymes for signal amplification.

In principle, when the cell target does not exist, cruciform DNA with biotin at three ends will hybridize with the sequence on the top of the arched DNA surface. Then, HRP labeled with streptavidin is immobilized by the streptavidin–biotin interaction, which can further catalyze the reaction of HQ and H$_2$O$_2$ on the electrode surface. In the presence of tumor cells, the cruciform DNA is released due to the affinity between the aptamer and the target, which effectively inhibits the sequent immobilization of HRP on the electrode surface, resulting in a weak electrical signal. Therefore, the electrochemical signal is negatively correlated with the concentration of the target (Scheme 1). In this strategy, AuNPs/VS$_2$ plays a crucial role of signal amplification (Figure S1). Moreover, it may also provide a solid scaffold for the immobilization of arch DNA and cruciform DNA, and the latter further provides a large number of HRP loading sites, enabling the enzyme-mediated signal amplification. Therefore, a dual signal amplification system was fabricated by this design.

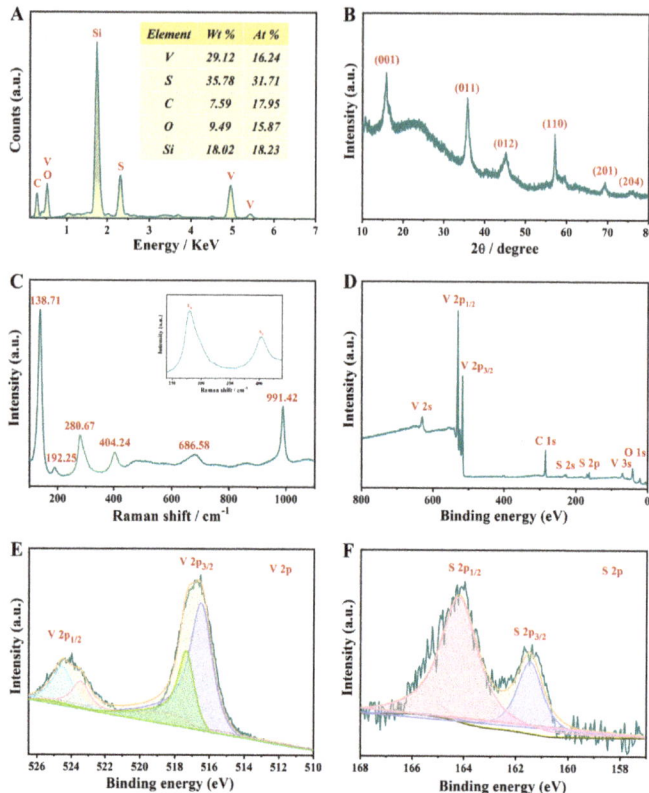

Figure 2. Characterization of VS$_2$ nanosheets: (**A**) EDS; (**B**) XRD; (**C**) Raman; (**D**) XPS. (**E,F**) show the amplified V 2p and S 2p zone in XPS.

The electrochemical characteristics on a series of modified electrodes were investigated by CV (Figure 3A,B) and EIS (Figure 3C,D). Firstly, the modification of VS$_2$ increases the electron transfer rate and the surface roughness of the electrode, resulting in a 1.3-fold increase in the electrochemical response (curve b) compared with bare GCE (curve a). Furthermore, the redox currents further increase by 27% upon the deposition of AuNPs on the modified electrode, giving AuNPs/VS$_2$/GCE (curve c). When the arch DNA is immobilized on the electrode surface (curve d), the negatively charged DNA strand hinders the electron transport of ferricyanide, and the redox currents decrease to a level similar to those on the bare electrode (curve a). After the treatment of blocking agent MCH (curve e), the non-specific binding sites on the electrode surface are blocked, and the electrochemical signal further decreases by 15%. With the modification of cruciform DNA (curve f) and target MCF-7 cells (curve g), the electrostatic repulsion and steric hindrance induced by the DNA strand and cells further passivate the electrode surface. The last step of modification is to immobilize HRP to the biotin-labeled cruciform DNA strand, and it shows the lowest electrochemical signal due to the low conductivity of proteins (curve h).

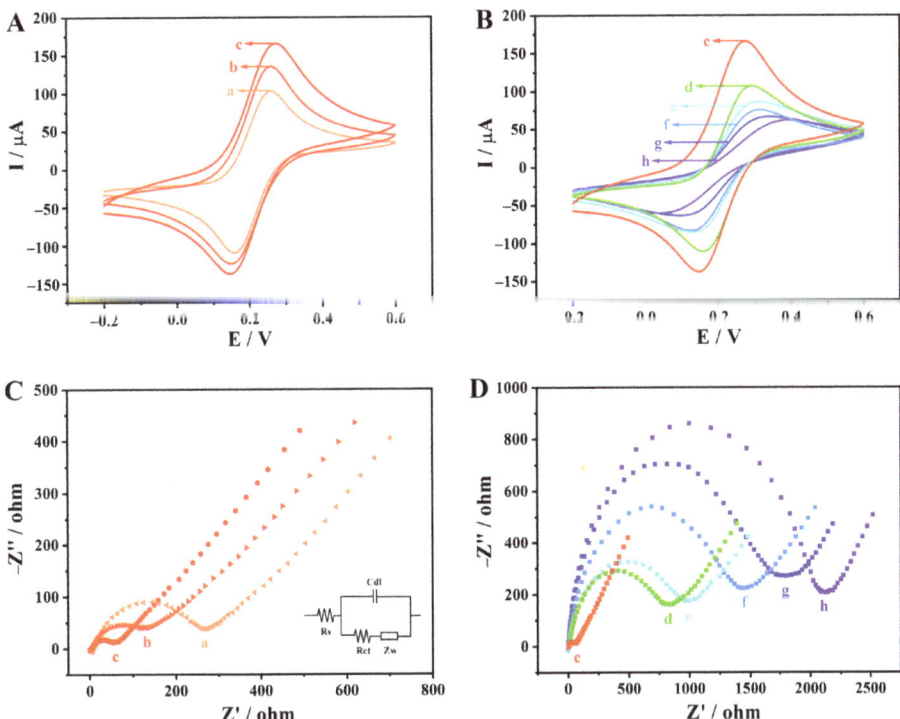

Figure 3. CV (**A,B**) and EIS (**C,D**) of different electrodes: (a) GCE; (b) VS$_2$/GCE; (c) AuNPs/VS$_2$/GCE; (d) arch DNA/AuNPs/VS$_2$/GCE; (e) MCH/arch DNA/AuNPs/VS$_2$/GCE; (f) cruciform DNA/MCH/arch DNA/AuNPs/VS$_2$/GCE; (g) target cell/cruciform DNA/MCH/arch DNA/AuNPs/VS$_2$/GCE; (h) HRP/target cell/cruciform DNA/MCH/arch DNA/AuNPs/VS$_2$/GCE. The inner illustration of (**C**) is the corresponding equivalent circuit diagram of the reaction system. Rct, Rs, Zw and Cdl in the circuit represent charge transfer resistance, solution resistance, Warburg impedance and electric double layer capacitance, respectively. Electrolyte: 0.1 M KCl containing 5 mM [Fe(CN)$_6$]$^{3-/4-}$.

Correspondingly, in the EIS plot (Figure 3C,D), the R_{ct} value of GCE is 260 Ω for bare GCE (curve a). After the electrodes are modified with VS$_2$ (curve b) and AuNPs/VS$_2$ (curve c), the R_{ct} value continues to decrease to 132 Ω and 67 Ω, respectively, proving the good conductivity of nanostructures. When arch DNA, MCH and cruciform DNA are added to the electrode surface in turn (curves d, e and f), the R_{ct} value increases greatly to 810 Ω, 960 Ω, and 1432 Ω, respectively, since both negatively charged DNA strands and MCH can reduce the electron transfer efficiency and increase the resistance of the system [35]. Finally, with the further immobilization of target cell MCF-7 and biotin-tagged HRP on the electrode surface (curve g and h), the R_{ct} value increases to 1710 Ω and 2053 Ω. The analysis results of EIS and CV are consistent, which proves the successful preparation of the sensor.

3.3. Optimization of Experimental Conditions

Under a cell concentration of 5000 cells/mL, the experimental conditions were optimized. Figure 4A shows the relationship of the DPV current and electrodeposition time for AuNPs. During the period of 10~25 s, the electrochemical response increases continuously, which corresponds to the stronger conductivity caused by AuNPs immobilized on the electrode. In the period of 25~70 s, the AuNP particles tend to be saturated, and the peak current basically remains stable. Therefore, 25 s is the best time for the electrodeposition of AuNPs.

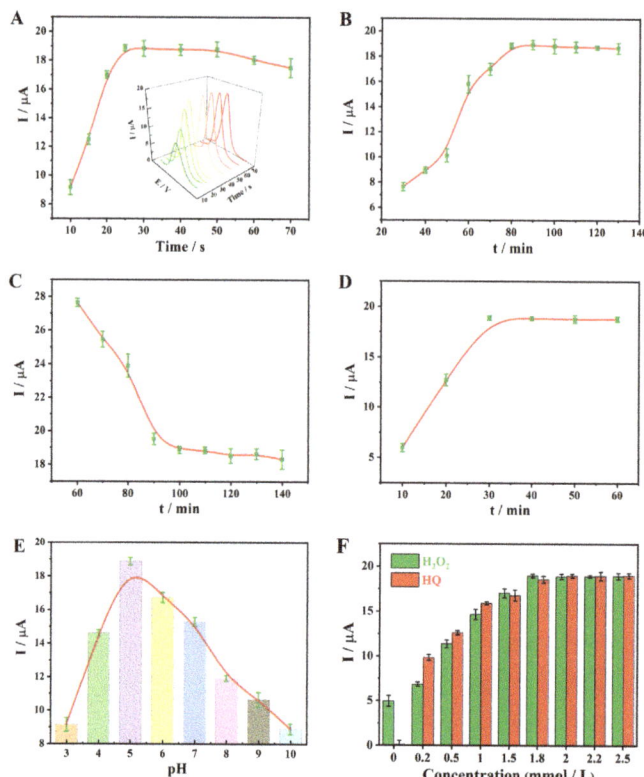

Figure 4. Optimization of experimental conditions: (**A**) deposition time of AuNPs; (**B**) incubation time of cruciform DNA; (**C**) incubation time of cells; (**D**) incubation time of HRP; (**E**) pH optimization; (**F**) concentration of H_2O_2 and HQ.

In addition to the deposition of Au NPs, the immobilization of the DNA strand is time-dependent. Figure 4B shows the DPV response after incubation cruciform DNA with a different time. When the incubation time is less than 80 min, the current continues to rise, indicating that the longer the incubation time is, the more HRP is bound. However, after 80 min, the current reaches stability and does not increase thereafter, due to the saturation of HRP loaded by cruciform DNA. The best incubation time for cruciform DNA is 80 min.

In addition, the cell incubation time is also an important parameter. As shown in Figure 4C, the cells gradually replace the cruciform DNA on arch DNA within 60~100 min, causing a reduction in the amount of immobilized cruciform DNA attached with HRP, as well as the enzyme catalyzed electrochemical signals. When the incubation time is more than 100 min, the peak current of DPV remains stable and does not decrease significantly, indicating that the cell incubation reaches equilibrium.

The incubation of biotin-labeled HRP can affect the performance of the sensor (Figure 4D). When the incubation time is less than 30 min, the immobilized amount of HRP increases with time, and the peak current increases gradually. After 30 min, the immobilized HRP on the electrode surface tends to be saturated. Therefore, the best time for HRP immobilization is 30 min. Since the pH and substrate concentrations are vital for HRP catalyzed reaction, this system was further optimized, obtaining an optimal pH of 5 (Figure 4E) and an optimal substrate concentration of 1.8 mmol/L (H_2O_2) and 2.0 mmol/L (HQ), respectively (Figure 4F).

3.4. Analysis Performance of Sensor

Under the above optimal experimental conditions, the sensor was used to detect different concentrations of MCF-7 cells. As shown in Figure 5A, the DPV signal gradually decreases with the increasing concentration of target cells. The DPV response is linearly correlated with the logarithm of MCF-7 cell concentration (Figure 5B, and 5B inset). The linear equation is I (µA) = 4.15 × log c (cells/mL) − 33.74, with a correlation coefficient R of 0.993. The linear range is 10 ~ 1 × 10^5 cells/mL, and the detection limit is 5 cells/mL (S/N = 3). In comparison, the linear range and limit of detection (LOD) for the reported MCF-7 sensors are listed in Table 1. The as-prepared MCF-7 sensor has a low LOD and a wide linear range among the cases, showing excellent electrochemical performances.

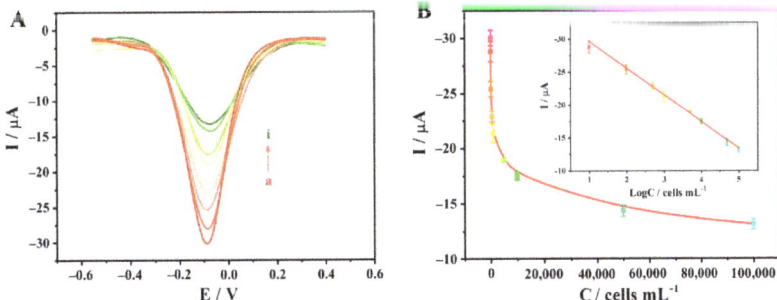

Figure 5. Detection performance of the sensor: (**A**) DPV curves of different concentrations of MCF-7, with the concentration of a~i: 0, 10, 10^2, 5 × 10^2, 1 × 10^3, 5 × 10^3, 1 × 10^4, 5 × 10^4, 1 × 10^5 cells/mL, respectively; (**B**) the relationship between the DPV current and the concentration of MCF-7. The inner illustration shows the linear relationship between the peak current of DPV and the logarithm of the MCF-7 cell concentration. The error bar represents the standard deviation of three measurements.

Table 1. Comparison between the constructed sensor and other sensors for detecting cells.

Detection Techniques	Experimental Methods	Linear Range (cell/mL)	LOD (cell/mL)	Ref.
EIS	Zr-MOF compound material	1 × 10^2 ~ 1 × 10^5	31	[36]
ICP-MS	Aptamer based bifunctional probe	2 × 10^2 ~ 1.2 × 10^4	81	[37]
Colorimetry	PH-AuPd-NPs combined 3D-rGO	50 ~ 1 × 10^7	32	[38]
DPV	AuNGs/MWCNT-NH$_2$	1 × 10^2 ~ 1 × 10^6	80	[39]
CC	DNA walker	0 ~ 5 × 10^2	47	[40]
ICP-MS	Magnetic bead binding anti-EpCAM	2 × 10^2 ~ 4 × 10^3	50	[41]
EIS	Clay-protein based nanocomposites	1.5 × 10^2 ~ 7.5 × 10^6	148	[42]
DPV	Branched chain peptide modified electrode interface	50 ~ 1 × 10^6	20	[43]
Fluorescence	aptamer-modified magnetic beads	10 ~ 1 × 10^5	5	[44]
DPV	BSA@Ag@Ir metallic-organic nanoclusters	3 ~ 3 × 10^6	1	[45]
DPV	Arch DNA, cruciform DNA, material signal amplification, enzyme amplification	10 ~ 1 × 10^5	5	This work

ICP-MS: inductively coupled plasma mass spectrometry.

3.5. Specificity, Reproducibility, Stability and Real Sample Analysis

The specificity of the sensor was investigated. In Figure 6A, the DPV responses to SGC-7901, HeLa, A549, L02 and MCF-7 cell suspensions with a concentration of 5000 cells/mL were tested, respectively. Only MCF-7 cells can significantly reduce the DPV signal, while in the presence of the other cells they exhibit a large electrochemical response, i.e., negligible cell attachment to the electrode interface. There is no significant difference in the current between a mixture of MCF-7 and L02 cell suspensions with the same concentrations and that of a pure MCF-7 cell suspension, which further proves that the prepared sensor has good specificity for MCF-7 cells.

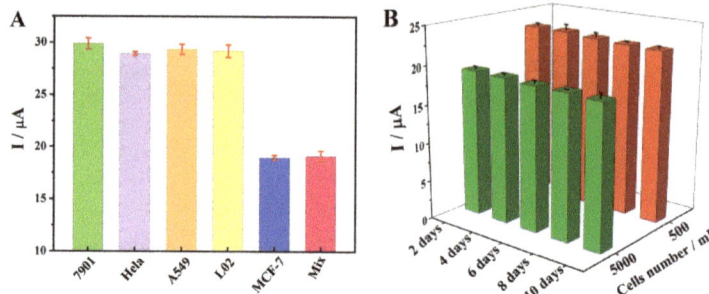

Figure 6. The specificity (**A**) and stability (**B**) of MCF-7 cell sensor.

Next, the reproducibility of the sensor is explored. Six parallel sensors were prepared to detect MCF-7 cells with a concentration of 500 cells/mL. The RSD of DPV peak current is 4.5%, indicating that the sensor has good reproducibility. In order to verify the storage stability, 10 electrodes were prepared in parallel and stored in a refrigerator at 4 °C for 10 days. According to the concentration of MCF-7 cells, they were divided into two groups: 500 cells/mL and 5000 cells/mL, with five electrodes in each group. The change of the DPV current was detected every two days (Figure 6B). There is no significant difference in the peak current between the two groups, indicating that the sensor has good stability.

In order to verify the application of the sensor in real samples, the recovery rates of MCF-7 in PBS and 10 times diluted whole-blood samples were tested, as shown in Table 2. For the concentration range of MCF-7 cells from 10 to 5×10^3 cells/mL, the recovery rates of MCF-7 spiked in PBS and diluted blood samples are 90.0~103.2% and 77.8~84.1%, respectively. The main reason for the low recovery rate in blood samples may be caused by many potential interferences such as red blood cells, white blood cells and high concentrated proteins in whole blood.

Table 2. Detection of MCF-7 in PBS and human whole-blood samples (n = 3).

Sample	Concentration (cells/mL)		Recovery Rate (%)
	Amount Added	Measured Value	
PBS	10	9	90.0
	100	92	92.0
	500	479	95.8
	1000	983	98.3
	2000	2063	103.2
	5000	4760	95.2
Blood sample	10	8	80.0
	100	83	83.0
	500	389	77.8
	1000	841	84.1

4. Conclusions

We have proposed a dual amplification strategy for the fabrication of a highly sensitive electrochemical biosensor for MCF-7 cells. In principle, AuNPs/VS$_2$ composites cannot only efficiently amplify the electrochemical signals due to their high conductivity, but also provide a solid scaffold for the hybridization of arch DNA and biotin-terminated cruciform DNA, as well as the following attachment of streptavidin-labeled HRP, which allows further enzyme catalyzed amplification. MCF-7 cells may competitively bind to the arch DNA and cause the release of cruciform DNA, which decreases the final amount of HRP immobilized on the electrode surface, thus reducing the electrochemical response by HRP catalysis. The DPV current is negatively correlated with the concentration of the target cells, with a linear range of 10 ~ 1 × 10^5 cells/mL, and a LOD of 5 cells/mL. In addition to good anti-interference ability to other types of cells, the biosensor may be applied for the detection of spiked cells in blood samples, suggesting its great applicability in the early diagnosis of breast cancer.

Supplementary Materials: The following are available online at https://www.mdpi.com/article/10.3390/bios11100378/s1, Figure S1: Signal amplification of nanocomposites: (A) Q-t curves of GCE and AuNPs/VS2/GCE, with Q-t1/2 curves of GCE and AuNPs/VS2/GCE in the inner illustration; (B) The DPV responses of HRP/target cell/cruciform DNA/MCH/arch-DNA structure/AuNPs/GCE (a) and HRP/target cell/cruciform DNA/MCH/arch-DNA structure/AuNPs/VS2/GCE (b). Figure S2: (A) Cytotoxicity test of arch DNA (green) and cruciform DNA (red); (B) Cruciform DNA electrophoresis. Lane 1–9: DNA1, DNA2, DNA3, DNA4, DNA1+DNA2, DNA2+DNA4, DNA1+DNA2+DNA3, DNA2+DNA3+DNA4, DNA1+DNA2+DNA3+DNA4. Table S1: DNA sequences. Table S2. List of instruments. Table S3: Experimental conditions and electrochemical parameters.

Author Contributions: Conceptualization, K.H., X.W. and H.J.; Data curation, J.Q., Y.W. and J.Z.; Formal analysis, Y.W.; Funding acquisition, K.H., X.W. and H.J.; Methodology, Y.W. and J.Z.; Writing—original draft, J.Q.; Writing—review & editing, H.J. All authors have read and agreed to the published version of the manuscript.

Funding: This work was funded by the National Natural Science Foundation of China (no. 92061121, 21974019, 82061148012, 82027806, and 22074130), the National Key Research & Development Program of China (2017YFA0205301), Primary Research & Development Plan of Jiangsu Province (BE2019716), Zhongyuan Thousand Talents Plan-Science and Technology Innovation Leading Talents Project (204200510030), Henan Provincial Science and Technology Innovation Team (No. C20150026), Nanhu Scholars Program of XYNU, and the Fundamental Research Funds for the Central Universities (KYCX20_0142).

Institutional Review Board Statement: Not applicable.

Informed Consent Statement: Not applicable.

Data Availability Statement: The data presented in this study are available in supplementary material.

Acknowledgments: This work is supported by the National Natural Science Foundation of China (no. 92061121, 21974019, 82061148012, 82027806, and 22074130), the National Key Research & Development Program of China (2017YFA0205301), Primary Research & Development Plan of Jiangsu Province (BE2019716), Zhongyuan Thousand Talents Plan-Science and Technology Innovation Leading Talents Project (204200510030), Henan Provincial Science and Technology Innovation Team (No. C20150026), Nanhu Scholars Program of XYNU, and the Fundamental Research Funds for the Central Universities (KYCX20_0142).

Conflicts of Interest: The authors declare no conflict of interest.

References

1. Wang, K.; He, M.-Q.; Zhai, F.-H.; He, R.-H.; Yu, Y.-L. A novel electrochemical biosensor based on polyadenine modified aptamer for label-free and ultrasensitive detection of human breast cancer cells. *Talanta* **2017**, *166*, 87–92. [CrossRef]
2. Li, T.; Fan, Q.; Liu, T.; Zhu, X.; Zhao, J.; Li, G. Detection of breast cancer cells specially and accurately by an electrochemical method. *Biosens. Bioelectron.* **2010**, *25*, 2686–2689. [CrossRef] [PubMed]
3. Dai, X.; Cheng, H.; Bai, Z.; Li, J. Breast Cancer Cell Line Classification and Its Relevance with Breast Tumor Subtyping. *J. Cancer* **2017**, *8*, 3131–3141. [CrossRef]
4. Sheng, Q.; Cheng, N.; Bai, W.; Zheng, J. Ultrasensitive electrochemical detection of breast cancer cells based on DNA-rolling-circle-amplification-directed enzyme-catalyzed polymerization. *Chem. Commun.* **2015**, *51*, 2114–2117. [CrossRef] [PubMed]
5. Liu, R.; Wang, Q.; Li, Q.; Yang, X.; Wang, K.; Nie, W. Surface plasmon resonance biosensor for sensitive detection of microRNA and cancer cell using multiple signal amplification strategy. *Biosens. Bioelectron.* **2017**, *87*, 433–438. [CrossRef]
6. Li, Y.; Huan, K.; Deng, D.; Tang, L.; Wang, J.; Luo, L. Facile Synthesis of ZnMn2O4@rGO Microspheres for Ultrasensitive Electrochemical Detection of Hydrogen Peroxide from Human Breast Cancer Cells. *ACS Appl. Mater. Interfaces* **2019**, *12*, 3430–3437. [CrossRef] [PubMed]
7. Bernsdorf, M.; Berthelsen, A.K.; Wielenga, V.T.; Kroman, N.; Teilum, D.; Binderup, T.; Tange, U.B.; Andersson, M.; Kjær, A.; Loft, A.; et al. Preoperative PET/CT in early-stage breast cancer. *Ann. Oncol.* **2012**, *23*, 2277–2282. [CrossRef]

8. Luo, Y.; Pan, Q.; Yang, H.; Peng, L.; Zhang, W.; Li, F. Fibroblast Activation Protein–Targeted PET/CT with 68Ga-FAPI for Imaging IgG4-Related Disease: Comparison to 18F-FDG PET/CT. *J. Nucl. Med.* **2021**, *62*, 266–271. [CrossRef]
9. Warner, E.; Plewes, D.B.; Hill, K.A.; Causer, P.A.; Zubovits, J.T.; Jong, R.A.; Cutrara, M.R.; DeBoer, G.; Yaffe, M.J.; Messner, S.J.; et al. Surveillance of BRCA1 and BRCA2 Mutation Carriers With Magnetic Resonance Imaging, Ultrasound, Mammography, and Clinical Breast Examination. *JAMA* **2004**, *292*, 1317–1325. [CrossRef]
10. Hananouchi, T.; Chen, Y.; Jerban, S.; Teramoto, M.; Ma, Y.; Dorthe, E.; Chang, E.; Du, J.; D'Lima, D. A Useful Combination of Quantitative Ultrashort Echo Time MR Imaging and a Probing Device for Biomechanical Evaluation of Articular Cartilage. *Biosensors* **2021**, *11*, 52. [CrossRef]
11. Galgano, S.; Viets, Z.; Fowler, K.; Gore, L.; Thomas, J.V.; McNamara, M.; McConathy, J. Practical Considerations for Clinical PET/MR Imaging. *Magn. Reson. Imaging Clin. N. Am.* **2017**, *25*, 281–296. [CrossRef] [PubMed]
12. Giesel, F.L.; Adeberg, S.; Syed, M.; Lindner, T.; Jiménez-Franco, L.D.; Mavriopoulou, E.; Staudinger, F.; Tonndorf-Martini, E.; Regnery, S.; Rieken, S.; et al. FAPI-74 PET/CT Using Either 18F-AlF or Cold-Kit 68Ga Labeling: Biodistribution, Radiation Dosimetry, and Tumor Delineation in Lung Cancer Patients. *J. Nucl. Med.* **2021**, *62*, 201–207. [CrossRef] [PubMed]
13. Galanzha, E.I.; Kim, J.-W.; Zharov, V.P. Nanotechnology-based molecular photoacoustic and photothermal flow cytometry platform forin-vivodetection and killing of circulating cancer stem cells. *J. Biophotonics* **2009**, *2*, 725–735. [CrossRef] [PubMed]
14. Mittal, S.; Kaur, H.; Gautam, N.; Mantha, A.K. Biosensors for breast cancer diagnosis: A review of bioreceptors, biotransducers and signal amplification strategies. *Biosens. Bioelectron.* **2017**, *88*, 217–231. [CrossRef] [PubMed]
15. Wang, Q.; Zou, L.; Yang, X.; Liu, X.; Nie, W.; Zheng, Y.; Cheng, Q.; Wang, K. Direct quantification of cancerous exosomes via surface plasmon resonance with dual gold nanoparticle-assisted signal amplification. *Biosens. Bioelectron.* **2019**, *135*, 129–136. [CrossRef] [PubMed]
16. Su, M.; Liu, H.; Ge, L.; Wang, Y.; Ge, S.; Yu, J.; Yan, M. Aptamer-Based electrochemiluminescent detection of MCF-7 cancer cells based on carbon quantum dots coated mesoporous silica nanoparticles. *Electrochim. Acta* **2014**, *146*, 262–269. [CrossRef]
17. Wang, X.; Cheng, S.; Wang, X.; Wei, L.; Kong, Q.; Ye, M.; Luo, X.; Xu, J.; Zhang, C.; Xian, Y. pH-Sensitive Dye-Based Nanobioplatform for Colorimetric Detection of Heterogeneous Circulating Tumor Cells. *ACS Sens.* **2021**, *6*, 1925–1932. [CrossRef]
18. Luo, J.; Liang, D.; Li, X.; Deng, L.; Wang, Z.; Yang, M. Aptamer-based photoelectrochemical assay for the determination of MCF-7. *Microchim. Acta* **2020**, *187*, 1–7. [CrossRef]
19. Huang, R.; Xi, Z.; He, N. Applications of aptamers for chemistry analysis, medicine and food security. *Sci. China Ser. B Chem.* **2015**, *58*, 1122–1130. [CrossRef]
20. Vajhadin, F.; Ahadian, S.; Travas-Sejdic, J.; Lee, J.; Mazloum-Ardakani, M.; Salvador, J.; Aninwene, G.E.; Bandaru, P.; Sun, W.; Khademhosseini, A. Electrochemical cytosensors for detection of breast cancer cells. *Biosens. Bioelectron.* **2020**, *151*, 111984. [CrossRef]
21. Lu, F.; Yang, L.; Hou, T.; Li, F. Label-free and "signal-on" homogeneous photoelectrochemical cytosensing strategy for ultrasensitive cancer cell detection. *Chem. Commun.* **2020**, *56*, 11126–11129. [CrossRef] [PubMed]
22. Zhu, D.; Liu, B.; Wei, G. Two-Dimensional Material-Based Colorimetric Biosensors: A Review. *Biosensors* **2021**, *11*, 259. [CrossRef] [PubMed]
23. Kasani, S.P.K.; Curtin, K.; Wu, N. A review of 2D and 3D plasmonic nanostructure array patterns: Fabrication, light management and sensing applications. *Nanophotonics* **2019**, *8*, 2065–2089. [CrossRef]
24. Wang, Y.-H.; Huang, K.-J.; Wu, X. Recent advances in transition-metal dichalcogenides based electrochemical biosensors: A review. *Biosens. Bioelectron.* **2017**, *97*, 305–316. [CrossRef]
25. Yu, D.; Pang, Q.; Gao, Y.; Wei, Y.; Wang, C.; Chen, G.; Du, F. Hierarchical flower-like VS2 nanosheets — A high rate-capacity and stable anode material for sodium-ion battery. *Energy Storage Mater.* **2018**, *11*, 1–7. [CrossRef]
26. Li, W.; Sari, H.M.K.; Li, X. Emerging Layered Metallic Vanadium Disulfide for Rechargeable Metal-Ion Batteries: Progress and Opportunities. *ChemSusChem* **2020**, *13*, 1172–1202. [CrossRef]
27. Xua, D.; Wanga, H.; Qiua, R.; Wangb, Q.; Maoa, Z.; Jiangc, Y.; Wanga, R.; Hea, B.; Gonga, Y.; Lib, D.; et al. Coupling of bowl-like VS2 nanosheet arrays and carbon nanofiber enables ultrafast Na+-Storage and robust flexibility for sodium-ion hybrid capacitors. *Energy Storage Mater.* **2020**, *28*, 91–100. [CrossRef]
28. Mikhaleva, N.S.; Visotin, M.A.; Kuzubov, A.A.; Popov, Z.I. VS2/Graphene Heterostructures as Promising Anode Material for Li-Ion Batteries. *J. Phys. Chem. C* **2017**, *121*, 24179–24184. [CrossRef]
29. Liu, Y.-Y.; Xu, L.; Guo, X.-T.; Lv, T.-T.; Pang, H. Vanadium sulfide based materials: Synthesis, energy storage and conversion. *J. Mater. Chem. A* **2020**, *8*, 20781–20802. [CrossRef]
30. Xie, X.-C.; Shuai, H.-L.; Wu, X.; Huang, K.-J.; Wang, L.-N.; Wang, R.-M.; Chen, Y. Engineering ultra-enlarged interlayer carbon-containing vanadium disulfide composite for high-performance sodium and potassium ion storage. *J. Alloy. Compd.* **2020**, *847*, 156288. [CrossRef]
31. Tian, L.; Zhang, Y.; Wang, L.; Geng, Q.; Liu, D.; Duan, L.; Wang, Y.; Cui, J. Ratiometric Dual Signal-Enhancing-Based Electrochemical Biosensor for Ultrasensitive Kanamycin Detection. *ACS Appl. Mater. Interfaces* **2020**, *12*, 52713–52720. [CrossRef]
32. Wang, M.; Chen, Y.; Cai, W.; Feng, H.; Du, T.; Liu, W.; Jiang, H.; Pasquarelli, A.; Weizmann, Y.; Wang, X. In situ self-assembling Au-DNA complexes for targeted cancer bioimaging and inhibition. *Proc. Natl. Acad. Sci. USA* **2020**, *117*, 308–316. [CrossRef] [PubMed]

33. Chen, Y.-X.; Huang, K.-J.; Lin, F.; Fang, L.-X. Ultrasensitive electrochemical sensing platform based on graphene wrapping SnO2 nanocorals and autonomous cascade DNA duplication strategy. *Talanta* **2017**, *175*, 168–176. [CrossRef]
34. He, P.; Yan, M.; Zhang, G.; Sun, R.; Chen, L.; An, Q.; Mai, L. Layered VS2 Nanosheet-Based Aqueous Zn Ion Battery Cathode. *Adv. Energy Mater.* **2017**, *7*, 1601920. [CrossRef]
35. Huang, L.; Deng, H.; Zhong, X.; Zhu, M.; Chai, Y.; Yuan, R.; Yuan, Y. Wavelength distinguishable signal quenching and enhancing toward photoactive material 3,4,9,10-perylenetetracarboxylic dianhydride for simultaneous assay of dual metal ions. *Biosens. Bioelectron.* **2019**, *145*, 111702. [CrossRef]
36. Li, Y.; Hu, M.; Huang, X.; Wang, M.; He, L.; Song, Y.; Jia, Q.; Zhou, N.; Zhang, Z.; Du, M. Multicomponent zirconium-based metal-organic frameworks for impedimetric aptasensing of living cancer cells. *Sens. Actuators B Chem.* **2020**, *306*, 127608. [CrossRef]
37. Yang, B.; Chen, B.; He, M.; Yin, X.; Xu, C.; Hu, B. Aptamer-Based Dual-Functional Probe for Rapid and Specific Counting and Imaging of MCF-7 Cells. *Anal. Chem.* **2018**, *90*, 2355–2361. [CrossRef] [PubMed]
38. Wang, H.; Zhou, C.; Sun, Y.; Jian, Y.; Kong, Q.; Cui, K.; Ge, S.; Yu, J. Polyhedral-AuPd nanoparticles-based dual-mode cytosensor with turn on enable signal for highly sensitive cell evaluation on lab-on-paper device. *Biosens. Bioelectron.* **2018**, *117*, 651–658. [CrossRef] [PubMed]
39. Yang, Y.; Fu, Y.; Su, H.; Mao, L.; Chen, M. Sensitive detection of MCF-7 human breast cancer cells by using a novel DNA-labeled sandwich electrochemical biosensor. *Biosens. Bioelectron.* **2018**, *122*, 175–182. [CrossRef]
40. Cai, S.; Chen, M.; Liu, M.; He, W.; Liu, Z.; Wu, D.; Xia, Y.; Yang, H.; Chen, J. A signal amplification electrochemical aptasensor for the detection of breast cancer cell via free-running DNA walker. *Biosens. Bioelectron.* **2016**, *85*, 184–189. [CrossRef]
41. Li, X.; Chen, B.; He, M.; Wang, H.; Xiao, G.; Yang, B.; Hu, B. Simultaneous detection of MCF-7 and HepG2 cells in blood by ICP-MS with gold nanoparticles and quantum dots as elemental tags. *Biosens. Bioelectron.* **2017**, *90*, 343–348. [CrossRef]
42. Yaman, Y.T.; Akbal, Ö.; Abaci, S. Development of clay-protein based composite nanoparticles modified single-used sensor platform for electrochemical cytosensing application. *Biosens. Bioelectron.* **2019**, *132*, 230–237. [CrossRef]
43. Liu, N.; Song, J.; Lu, Y.; Davis, J.J.; Gao, F.; Luo, X. Electrochemical Aptasensor for Ultralow Fouling Cancer Cell Quantification in Complex Biological Media Based on Designed Branched Peptides. *Anal. Chem.* **2019**, *91*, 8334–8340. [CrossRef] [PubMed]
44. Shenab, C.; Zhongb, L.; Xiongab, L.; Liub, C.; Yuc, L.; Chuab, X.; Luoab, X.; Zhaob, M.; Liuab, B. A novel sandwich-like cytosensor based on aptamers-modified magnetic beads and carbon dots/cobalt oxyhydroxide nanosheets for circulating tumor cells detection. *Sens. Actuators B Chem.* **2021**, *331*, 129399. [CrossRef]
45. Shen, H.; Liu, L.; Yuan, Z.; Liu, Q.; Li, B.; Zhang, M.; Tang, H.; Zhang, J.; Zhao, S. Novel cytosensor for accurate detection of circulating tumor cells based on a dual-recognition strategy and BSA@Ag@Ir metallic-organic nanoclusters. *Biosens. Bioelectron.* **2021**, *179*, 113102. [CrossRef] [PubMed]

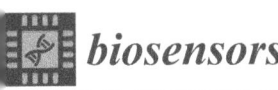

Article

Stability Assessment of Four Chimeric Proteins for Human Chagas Disease Immunodiagnosis

Paola Alejandra Fiorani Celedon [1], Leonardo Maia Leony [2], Ueriton Dias Oliveira [1], Natália Erdens Maron Freitas [2], Ângelo Antônio Oliveira Silva [2], Ramona Tavares Daltro [2], Emily Ferreira Santos [2], Marco Aurélio Krieger [1,3,4], Nilson Ivo Tonin Zanchin [3] and Fred Luciano Neves Santos [2,4,*]

1. Molecular Biology Institute of Paraná, Curitiba, Paraná 81350-010, Brazil; paolafc@ibmp.org.br (P.A.F.C.); u.doliveira@ibmp.org.br (U.D.O.); marco.krieger@fiocruz.br (M.A.K.)
2. Gonçalo Moniz Institute, Oswaldo Cruz Foundation, Salvador, Bahia 40296-710, Brazil; leonardo.leony@fiocruz.br (L.M.L.); natalia.erdens@fiocruz.br (N.E.M.F.); angelo.oliveira@fiocruz.br (Â.A.O.S.); ramona.daltro@fiocruz.br (R.T.D.); emily.santos@fiocruz.br (E.F.S.)
3. Carlos Chagas Institute, Oswaldo Cruz Foundation, Curitiba, Paraná 81350-010, Brazil; nilson.zanchin@fiocruz.br
4. Integrated Translational Program in Chagas Disease from Fiocruz (Fio-Chagas), Vice Presidency of Research and Biological Collections, Oswaldo Cruz Foundation, Rio de Janeiro, Rio de Janeiro 21040-900, Brazil
* Correspondence: fred.santos@fiocruz.br; Tel.: +55-(71)-99390-3004

Abstract: The performance of an immunoassay relies on antigen-antibody interaction; hence, antigen chemical stability and structural integrity are paramount for an efficient assay. We conducted a functional, thermostability and long-term stability analysis of different chimeric antigens (IBMP), in order to assess effects of adverse conditions on four antigens employed in ELISA to diagnose Chagas disease. ELISA-based immunoassays have served as a model for biosensors development, as both assess molecular interactions. To evaluate thermostability, samples were heated and cooled to verify heat-induced denaturation reversibility. In relation to storage stability, the antigens were analyzed at 25 °C at different moments. Long-term stability tests were performed using eight sets of microplates sensitized. Antigens were structurally analyzed through circular dichroism (CD), dynamic light scattering, SDS-PAGE, and functionally evaluated by ELISA. Data suggest that IBMP antigens are stable, over adverse conditions and for over a year. Daily analysis revealed minor changes in the molecular structure. Functionally, IBMP-8.2 and IBMP-8.3 antigens showed reactivity towards anti-*T. cruzi* antibodies, even after 72 h at 25 °C. Long-term stability tests showed that all antigens were comparable to the control group and all antigens demonstrated stability for one year. Data suggest that the antigens maintained their function and structural characteristics even in adverse conditions, making them a sturdy and reliable candidate to be employed in future in vitro diagnostic tests applicable to different models of POC devices, such as modern biosensors in development.

Keywords: Chagas disease; immunoassays; chimeric proteins; stability

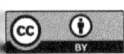

1. Introduction

Chagas disease is a deadly, neglected, tropical infection caused by the hemoflagellate parasite *Trypanosoma cruzi*. According to the World Health Organization, 5.7 million individuals are infected by the parasite, resulting in 7500 deaths annually, mostly in the continental Western Hemisphere, resulting in a massive disease burden in the 22 endemic countries [1]. The parasite can be transmitted through several pathways, such as by contact with excrements from infected triatomine bugs (hematophagous insects of the Triatominae family), consumption of contaminated beverages and food, from mother-to-child during pregnancy, whole blood or blood derivatives transfusion, tissue and organ transplantation and through laboratory work accidents [2].

Two distinct phases occur during the natural course of Chagas disease progression. The initial acute phase is characterized as an unspecific oligosymptomatic febrile illness.

Infected individuals present high parasitemia, which enables the parasitological diagnosis, based on the direct visualization of the parasite in a thick blood smear. The acute phase lasts for 2–3 months after initial infection. This is followed by the gradual resolution of the clinical manifestations (when present) and the start of the lifelong chronic phase, characterized by an intermittent or absent parasitemia, as well as high levels of IgG anti-*T. cruzi* antibodies [2]. As such, direct methods are unacceptably accurate as diagnostic methods in the chronic stage of the disease, thus, in vitro diagnostics (IVD) based on indirect immunoassays are overwhelmingly recommended. Indirect IVD methods are based on the detection of specific antibodies produced against a certain pathogen, such as indirect immunofluorescence (IIF), indirect hemagglutination (IHA), rapid diagnostic tests (RDT) and enzyme-linked immunosorbent assay (ELISA). Such serological methods rely on the interaction between the antibodies from the patient and epitopes from the pathogen antigen, as such, the structural integrity of those antigens is paramount for efficient antibody binding. Furthermore, the stability of the antigens over time and different environmental conditions must be taken into consideration. In a laboratory setting, the shelf and storage lifespan can be determinant when choosing the appropriate reagent for the routine and when point-of-care testing is being considered, an antigen must retain its structural integrity over a prolonged time, despite significant temperature variations, as can be expected between storage and transportation.

Among the available commercial IVD tests to identify chronic Chagas disease, ELISA and RDT are the most used due to their low cost and overall efficiency. However, these methodologies regularly present inconsistent performance, which is attributed to various distinct reasons, such as the chosen capture antigens [3], the varying degree of immune responses against the infection [4,5], *T. cruzi* high genetic and phenotypic intraspecific diversity [6] and variation in disease prevalence [7,8]. Accordingly, the World Health Organization (WHO) recommends the use of two different serological tests in parallel to diagnose Chagas disease in humans [9]. The use of chimeric proteins, composed of conserved immunodominant, and are tandemly repeated sequences of several different antigens of *T. cruzi*, can be a strategy to address the inconsistent performances of IVD tests [10–12]. This strategy can also address issues commonly attributed to recombinant proteins, such as the lower sensitivity in comparison to lysates or native antigen mixtures, which is attributed to a lower epitope diversity. The use of chimeric proteins in IVD simultaneously addresses the lack of reproducible performance parameters, while increasing both sensitivity and specificity, as a result of the greater diversity of distinct and conserved immunodominant epitopes, from numerous antigens, which are presented in these proteins. Chimeric proteins have also been employed in IVD [13–15] or as a vaccine [16,17] for other infectious diseases. Considering the predicaments herein set forth, our group expressed four *T. cruzi* chimeric proteins, called IBMP-8.1, IBMP-8.2, IBMP-8.3 and IBMP-8.4 (Molecular Biology Institute of Paraná—IBMP in Portuguese acronym), and assessed their performance in diagnosis chronic Chagas disease in dogs [18,19] and humans, from several endemic and non-endemic settings from Brazil [20], Argentina, Paraguay, Bolivia [21] and Spain [22].

The ability of immunoassays to detect specific antibodies depends on the spatial distribution and availability of epitopes on the solid phase. Although peptides sequences with conformational preferences have been shown to be preferentially recognized by antibodies against native protein epitopes, some evidence supports the idea that IBMP antigens are composed of linear epitopes [10]. Aggregate formation, degradation, or even conformation changes can lead to the impairment of antigen-antibody detection, caused by hidden or folded epitopes, hinder antigen accessibility, thereby leading to misdiagnosis. However, it is not clear whether these conditions, which are often the result of improper storage and handling, could impact the assay's performance when chimeric proteins composed of linear epitopes are employed as solid-phase antigens.

Likewise, due to IVD tests tendency to evolve towards automated and miniaturized microfluidic systems, it is pertinent to obtain data regarding the feasibility of novel molecules towards integrated IVD devices. Protein structural conformation, protein-protein interaction and stability assessment are paramount for an efficient immunoassay, whether it is applied in an ELISA system or microfluidic devices. Recently, the IBMP molecules performance profile for chronic Chagas disease diagnosis was similar to that of an impedimetric immunosensor using dual screen-printed carbon electrode [19], although these interactions in turn occurs mostly in liquid phase-like mode.

In this work, in order to evaluate the outcome of linking several epitopes separated by artificially designed spacers, we conducted a functional and structural analysis of four chimeric antigens for chronic Chagas disease in vitro diagnosis. We also assessed the impact of different antigen buffers and adverse environmental conditions on the performance of the immunoassays. Bearing in mind that the formation of secondary structures, dimerization and agglutination negatively impacts the performance of an indirect immunoassay from exploring linear epitopes, and that antigens are the main gear driving indirect serological methods, the analysis regarding an antigen's behavior at different environmental conditions, temperatures and buffers paves the way towards a robust antigen preparation for a reliable and biosensor.

2. Materials and Methods

2.1. Study Design

The study was carried out using both dissolved and adsorbed antigens (Figure 1). To stringently evaluate the extent of structural perturbations in different environmental conditions, thermic and long-term stability at 4 °C was analyzed. Initially, samples were heated up to 85 °C and cooled to 4 °C to verify the reversibility or irreversibility of heat-induced denaturation (time exposure in each temperature: 1 min, 10 min and 20 min). Therefore, samples were taken before, and after, the tests and analyzed by circular dichroism (CD), dynamic light scattering (DLS), sodium dodecyl sulfate-polyacrylamide gel electrophoresis (SDS-PAGE) and enzyme-linked immunosorbent assay (ELISA). With respect to storage stability of soluble antigens at room temperature (25 °C), we analyzed the samples at time zero (control) and aliquots were drawn out every 24 h for 72 h. Antigen structure was analyzed by CD, DLS, SDS-PAGE, and functionally assed through ELISA. Long-term stability tests at 4 °C were performed over 1 year (Figure 1). Accordingly, eight sets of microplates were sensitized with IBMP antigens and stored at 4 °C in hermetically sealed storage bags with desiccant. Similarly, eight sets of T. cruzi-positive and negative sera were aliquoted and stored at −20 °C until analysis functional and structural assessment through ELISA.

2.2. IBMP Protein Expression and Purification

Antigen sequence selection (Table 1), gene construction and recombinant expression were described in Santos et al. [10]. Briefly, T. cruzi synthetic genes were subcloned into the pET28a vector (Novagen, Madison, WI, USA) and expressed as soluble proteins in Escherichia coli BL21-Star (DE3) cells grown in LB medium supplemented with 0.5 µM isopropyl-β-D-1-thiogalactopyranoside (IPTG). The antigens were purified by affinity and ion-exchange chromatography using columns and chromatographers supplied by GE Healthcare. Finally, purified proteins were quantified using a fluorometric assay (Qubit 2.0, Invitrogen Technologies, Carlsbad, CA, USA).

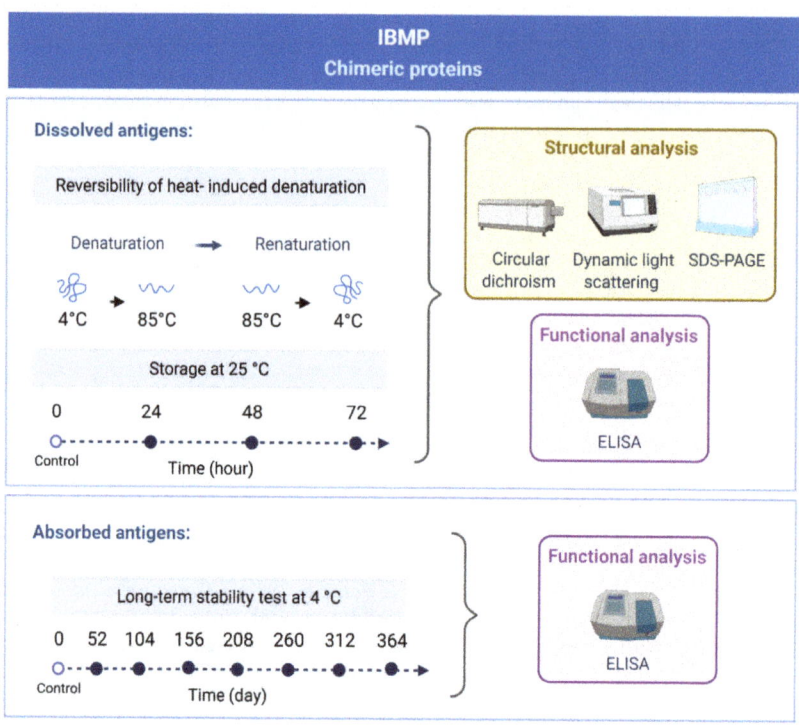

Figure 1. Flowchart of the study design for evaluating the stability of dissolved and absorbed IBMP chimeric proteins by using functional (ELISA) and structural (CD, DLS, SDS-PAGE) analysis.

Table 1. Constitution of the IBMP chimeric recombinant proteins.

Chimeric Antigen	Sequence Name	Amino Acid Range	Gene Bank Sequence ID
IBMP-8.1	Trans-sialidase 60S ribosomal protein L19 Trans-sialidase Surface antigen 2 (CA-2)	747–774 218–238 1435–1449 276–297	XP_820062.1 XP_820995.1 XP_813586.1 XP_813516.1
IBMP-8.2	Antigen, partial Surface antigen 2 (CA-2) Calpain cysteine peptidase	13–73 166–220 31–97	ACM47959.1 XP_818927.1 XP_804989.1
IBMP-8.3	Trans-sialidase Flagellar repetitive antigen protein 60S ribosomal protein L19 Surface antigen 2 (CA-2)	710–754 15–56 236–284 279–315	XP_813237.1 AAA30177.1 XP_808122.1 XP_813516.1
IBMP-8.4	Shed-acute-phase-antigen Kinetoplastid membrane protein KMP-11 Trans-sialidase Flagellar repetitive antigen protein Trans-sialidase Surface antigen 2 (CA-2) Flagellar repetitive antigen protein 60S ribosomal protein L19 Microtubule-associated protein	681–704 76–92 1436–1449 20–47 740–759 276–298 1–68 218–238 421–458	CAA40511.1 XP_810488.1 XP_813586.1 AAA30177.1 XP_820062.1 XP_813516.1 AAA30197.1 XP_820995.1 XP_809567.1

2.3. Gel Electrophoresis

Samples (1 µg) were resuspended in loading buffer, subjected to electrophoresis in SDS–PAGE [23] (8 × 9 cm and 0.75 mm thick, 12% polyacrylamide) and stained with Coomassie brilliant blue-250 for visualization. SDS-PAGE was used to evaluate the protein degradation of soluble antigens during analysis.

2.4. Circular Dichroism (CD) Measurements

To further evaluate thermal impact over structural content and conformation of IBMP antigens, far-UV CD spectra were assessed on a CD spectrophotometer, (Jasco J-815, Tokyo, Japan), equipped with a Peltier type CD/FL cell thermoelectric sample holder (Jasco, Tokyo, Japan). Samples were analyzed at 0.2 mg/mL in a 1-mm path length quartz cuvette. Each spectroscopic readout represented the average of four continuously acquired scans. All readouts were rectified considering the buffer background noise. Each scan within 193–260 or 202–260 nm range was acquired through a scanning rate of 100 nm/min, 0.5 nm data pitch, 1 nm bandwidth, and 1 s of data integration time. The results were expressed in molar ellipticity $[\theta]_\lambda$ (deg × cm^2 × dmol^{-1}) and shifts at 208–222 nm and 215 nm were used to assess α-, and β-structural content, respectively. Protein secondary structure analysis was performed using the Dichroweb platform.

2.5. Dynamic Light Scattering (DLS)

In order to determine the hydrodynamic radius (Rh) and polydispersity, DLS measurements were undertaken utilizing a DynaPro NanoStar Dynamic Light Scattering analyzer (Wyatt Technology Corp., Santa Barbara, CA, USA), equipped with a Ga-As laser (120 mW), operating at a wavelength of 658 nm. Protein samples were placed in a 1-mm^2 quartz cuvette and measurements were performed at RT (22–25 °C). Data analysis was carried out using the software Dynamics v.7.1.7.16.

2.6. Clinical Specimens and Indirect ELISA

Anonymized human sera samples from individuals infected (n = 46) or non-infected (n = 46) with *T. cruzi* were obtained from the Chagas Disease Reference Laboratory (Aggeu Magalhães Institute; Oswaldo Cruz Foundation, Pernambuco, Brazil) and used to assess the reactivity of IBMP antigens associated with the three different conditions (Figure 1). Sample characterization was based on the concordance between two distinct serological tests for Chagas disease, as recommended by the World Health Organization [9]. Assays were performed according to the procedure described previously [10]. Briefly, IBMP antigens were diluted at 12.5 ng (IBMP-8.2) and 25.0 ng (IBMP-8.1, IBMP-8.3 and IBMP-8.4) in carbonate buffer (0.05 M, pH 9.6), then 96-well microplates (Nunc, Roskilde, Denmark) were coated with 100 µL per well and subsequently blocked with Well Champion reagent (Kem-En-Tec, Taastrup, Denmark) according to the manufacturer's instructions. Sera samples were pre-diluted at 1:100 in 0.05 M phosphate-buffered saline (PBS; pH 7.2) and 100 µL was transferred to each well. After incubation at 37 °C for 60 min, the microplates were washed with PBS-0.05% Tween 20 (PBS-T). HRP-conjugated goat anti-human IgG (Bio-Manguinhos, FIOCRUZ, Rio de Janeiro, Brazil) was diluted in PBS at 1:40,000, and then 100 µL was transferred to each well and incubated for 30 min at 37 °C. Following the incubation and washing, 100 µL of TMB substrate solution (tetramethyl-benzidine; Kem-En-Tec, Taastrup, Denmark) was added and incubated at room temperature for 10 min in the dark. Finally, the reaction was stopped with 50 µL of 3 N H_2SO_4, and the optical density was measured at 450 nm in a Multiskan® FC microplate spectrophotometer (Thermo Scientific™, Ratastie, Finland).

2.7. Data Analysis

Geometric mean ± SD calculation was measured for all variables. In order to verify data normality, the Shapiro-Wilk test was performed, followed by Student's T test. Whenever data variance homogeneity assumption couldn't be confirmed, the Wilcoxon signed-ranks test was employed. All statistical significance analyses had a two-tailed distribution and a *p*-value under 5% was considered significant ($p < 0.05$). Regression curve analysis was performed for each temperature condition using positive/negative (P/N) ratio values and protein exposure period for each thermal reading point. ELISA reactivity data at different thermal conditions were subjected to statistical analysis employing student's t-test to assess significance level. Cut-off value analysis was defined by the largest distance from the diagonal line of the receiver operating characteristic curve (ROC) (sensitivity $\times$ (1-specificity)) to identify the optimal ELISA OD value that best differentiates between negative and positive samples. The confidence interval (CI) was developed to address the proportion estimates precision with a confidence level of 95%. Data were examined using GraphPad Prism version 8 (San Diego, CA, USA).

3. Results

3.1. Reversibility of Heat-Induced Denaturation

Since changes in CD spectra and light scattering may reflect structural shifts of the molecules, we previously characterized the IBMP chimeric antigens by these methodologies to determine their typical conformation under different buffer compositions [10]. On that occasion, 50 mM carbonate-bicarbonate buffer pH 9.6 was shown to be the most appropriate buffer system for reducing protein aggregation, while maintaining the original conformation. Now, we demonstrate that when soluble in carbonate buffer, the IBMP antigens are very stable, and even after some degradation under temperature effect, little of their diagnostic capacity is lost. By monitoring CD spectra of the 4 chimeric proteins, it could be seen that denaturation-renaturation by rapid thermal stress (from 4 °C to 85 °C to 4 °C) did not cause changes relative to the original conformation for antigens IBMP-8.1, IBMP-8.2 and IBMP-8.4 (Figure 2A,E,M). Whereas, IBMP-8.3 seems to keep an unfolded conformation after heat-denaturation (Figure 2I).

In the case of IBMP-8.2, the CD signals of pre- and post-heating are very similar, but the DLS analysis shows that it has aggregated as observed by the increase in the hydrodynamic radius. There is almost no degradation, which can be visualized by the analysis by electrophoresis on polyacrylamide gels (Figure 2C,G,K,O). Despite the denaturing conditions, all antigens continue to be recognized by anti-*T. cruzi* antibodies (Figure 2D,H,L,P), suggesting that individual epitopes remained competent for antibody interaction. Individual data points of reversibility of heat-induced denaturation evaluation are available in the Supplementary Materials, Table S1.

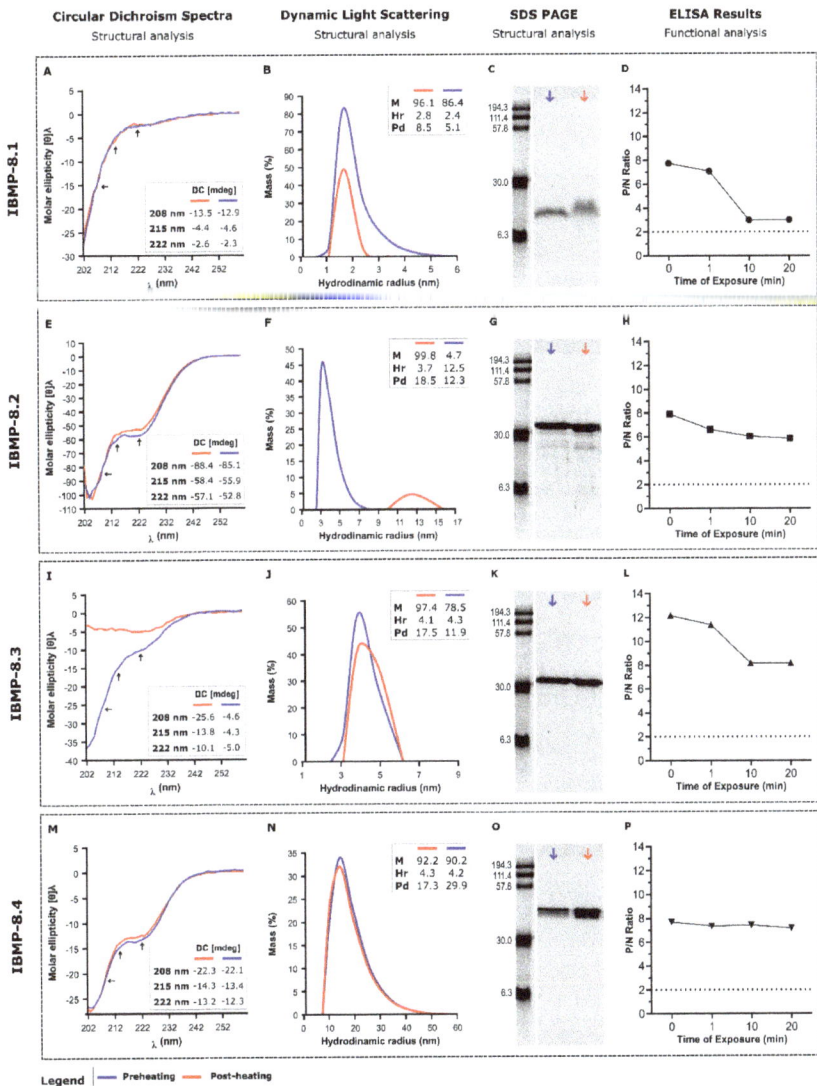

Figure 2. Evaluation of heat-induced denaturation reversibility for the IBMP recombinant chimeric proteins by CD, DLS, SDS-PAGE and sera reactivity by ELISA. CD (Circular dichroism); Hr (Hydrodynamic radius); M (%mass); min (Minute); nm (Nanometer); Pd (Polydispersity); P/N ratio (Positive/negative ratio). Boxes in (**A,E,I,M**) indicate the values of CD signal intensity at 208, 215 and 222 nm. Boxes in (**B,F,J,N**) indicate the values of %mass, hydrodynamic radius and polydispersity. (**C,G,K,O**) are the SDS-PAGE images of the antigens after the treatments. (**D,H,L,P**) shows the reactivity of the antigens in ELISA assay after the heat treatment.

3.2. Storage Stability at 25 °C

Daily analysis of the short-term assay revealed CD spectra highly similar to the original for the four proteins, indicating no changes in the conformation. The sudden increase of hydrodynamic radius (Hr) for IBMP-8.1 could represent an aggregation of the antigen while the Hr of the others remains similar to the original (Figure 3B,F,J,N). With respect to polydispersity, IBMP-8.1 seems to form homogenous aggregates and the reduced polydispersity of 8–4 at the 72 h time point may be due to degradation (Figure 3B). Gels show that IBMP-8.1 (Figure 3C) and IBMP-8.2 (Figure 3G) can hold most integrity until 72 h upon exposure to 25 °C in solution. In turn, IBMP-8.3 (Figure 3K) and IBMP-8.4 (Figure 3O) suffered severe degradation after 48 h. Although protein degradation was seen on the gels (not determined sizes), CD spectra did not change significantly at the 72 h time point for IBMP-8.3 and IBMP-8.4. The CD signal of these samples may be provided by the protein fragments still present in the samples. Functionally, IBMP-8.2 (Figure 3H) and IBMP-8.3 (Figure 3L) antigens showed reactivity to anti-*T. cruzi* antibodies, even 72 h after the beginning of the analyzes. Contrarily, IBMP-8.1 (Figure 3D) and IBMP-8.4 (Figure 3P) antigens have gradually lost their reactivity in the ELISA assays after 72 h. Individual data points of storage stability at 25 °C evaluation are available in the Supplementary Materials, Table S2.

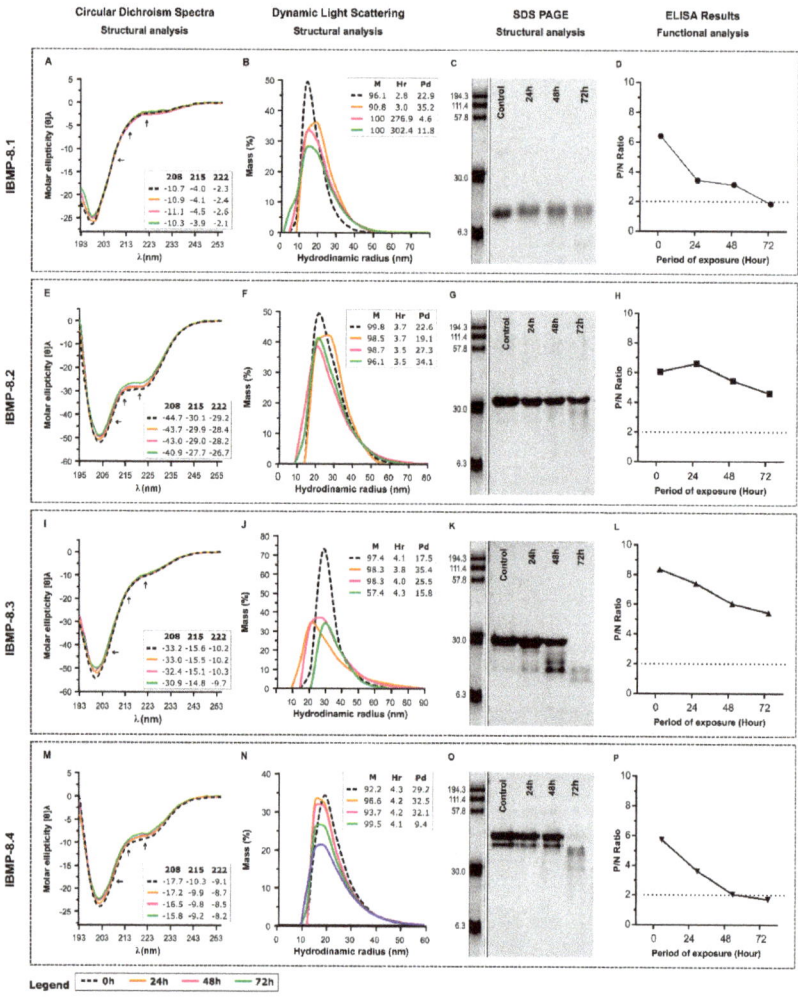

Figure 3. Evaluation of storage stability at 25 °C for IBMP recombinant chimeric proteins by CD, DLS, SDS-PAGE and sera reactivity by ELISA. DC (Circular dichroism); h (hours); Hr (hydrodynamic radius); M (%mass); nm (Nanometer); P/N ratio (Positive/negative ratio). Boxes in (**A,E,I,M**) indicate the values of CD signal intensity at 208, 215 and 222 nm. Boxes in (**B,F,J,N**) indicate the values of %mass, hydrodynamic radius and polydispersity. (**C,G,K,O**) are the SDS-PAGE images in the times described. (**D,H,L,P**) represent the reactivity of the antigens in ELISA assay after exposure time.

3.3. Long-Term Stability Analysis at 4 °C

Long-term stability tests at 4 °C were performed using eight points of ELISA over 1 year (Figure 4). The P/N ratio of all IBMP chimeric proteins was comparable to that found for the control group (time 0), therefore, the ratio did not modify after 364 days. Exceptions for IBMP-8.1 and IBMP-8.3 antigens after 312, and 260 days, respectively. In these cases, P/N ratio slightly declined, but remained above the cut-off (Figure 4A; Individual data points are available in the Supplementary Materials, Table S3). Overall, all absorbed proteins have shown stability over 1 year. Similar results were observed when accuracy diagnostic was assessed. Considering the overlap of 95% CI values, no significant difference in accuracy was observed among all eight analysis points for the four antigens (Figure 4B).

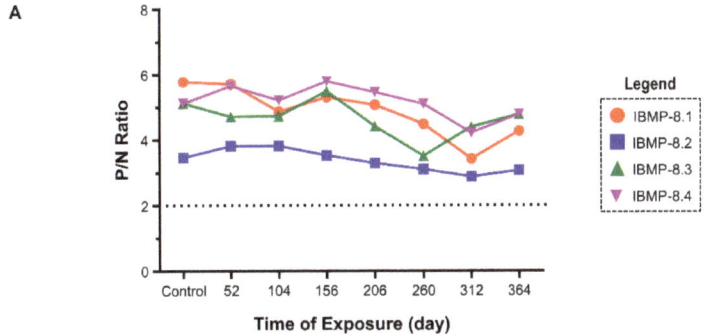

B

	Accuracy values (95%CI)			
	IBMP-8.1	IBMP-8.2	IBMP-8.3	IBMP-8.4
Control	100 (96.0-100)	100 (96.0-100)	100 (96.0-100)	100 (96.0-100)
52 days	95.7 (89.3-98.3)	93.5 (86.5-97.0)	92.4 (85.1-96.3)	94.6 (87.9-97.7)
104 days	95.7 (89.3-98.3)	92.4 (85.1-96.3)	93.5 (86.5-97.0)	95.7 (89.3-98.3)
156 days	95.7 (89.3-98.3)	93.5 (86.5-97.0)	93.5 (86.5-97.0)	96.7 (90.8-98.9)
206 days	96.7 (90.8-98.9)	93.5 (86.5-97.0)	96.7 (90.8-98.9)	97.8 (92.4-99.4)
260 days	92.4 (85.1-96.3)	92.4 (85.1-96.3)	92.4 (85.1-96.3)	92.4 (85.1-96.3)
312 days	92.4 (85.1-96.3)	92.4 (85.1-96.3)	92.4 (85.1-96.3)	94.6 (87.9-97.7)
364 days	92.4 (85.1-96.3)	92.4 (85.1-96.3)	93.5 (86.5-97.0)	93.5 (86.5-97.0)

Figure 4. Stability of IBMP chimeric proteins over 1 year. (**A**) Ratio of positive to negative (P/N) serum reactivity in indirect ELISA; (**B**) Accuracy values for each point of analysis.

4. Discussion

The high accuracy of IBMP (-8.1, -8.2, -8.3 and -8.4) chimeric antigens in diagnosing chronic Chagas disease, both in endemic and non-endemic settings has been established in previous studies [10,19–22,24–27]. However, the stability of these molecules under different stress situations was not yet known. Here, we explored the structural stability of these four antigens in different conditions using CD and DLS to gain information on the level of alterations that might take place on their structure and state of oligomerization and aggregation, respectively. Moreover, protein degradation and functional analysis have been carried out by SDS-PAGE, and indirect ELISA, respectively. Although their performance could be determined by any immunological technique, using microtiter plates, beads, nanosensors and others [28,29]. We also evaluated the stability of absorbed antigens in microplates for one year. The results obtained allow us to infer that all chimeric antigens are highly stable, preserving their functionality in immunoassays, even after exposure to extreme conditions.

Previously, our group characterized the secondary structure content and solubility of these IBMP chimeric antigen in different buffering agents: 50 mM carbonate-bicarbonate, pH 9.6; 50 mM sodium phosphate, pH 7.5; and 50 mM MES ([2-(n-morpholino) ethanesulfonic acid], pH 5.5) [10]. Those studies have demonstrated that IBMP-8.1 and IBMP-8.3 proteins predominantly comprised random coil as verified by neutral CD values between 215 and 240 nm and negative values at about 200 nm. On the other hand, CD spectra of IBMP-8.2 and IBMP-8.4 proteins exhibited a negative minimum at ~203 nm and shoulder at ~220 nm. The intensity of the CD signal at ~220 nm indicates that, in addition to random coil, IBMP-8.2 and IBMP-8.4 present also a certain content of α-helices. No conformational changes were observed in IBMP-8.1 and IBMP-8.3 coil proteins upon solubilization in different buffering agents. However, CD spectra of IBMP-8.3 and IBMP-8.4 proteins showed a slight shift to longer wavelengths upon solubilization in acidic pH, indicating changes in secondary structure content. With respect to DLS data, all proteins presented less polydisperse values (<20%) in 50 mM carbonate-bicarbonate (pH 9.6) when compared to other buffers tested. These data indicate that all proteins can be influenced by the environment. Therefore, 50 mM carbonate-bicarbonate (pH 9.6) buffer system was chosen to carry out the present study.

The chosen buffer alone conserved epitopes even during long lasting storage. The use of stabilizing compounds, which increases costs and offers interference, especially with downstream applications, is a common issue regarding antigen and antibodies storage. The reduced intrinsic structure of our molecules makes them ideal for various methodologies, where negative interferences are caused by detergents and reducing or chaotropic agents.

CD spectra on the reversibility of heat-induced denaturation assessment showed that only IBMP-8.3 chimeric protein underwent a strong change in CD signal, assuming an unfolded conformation after heating. For other proteins (IBMP-8.1, IBMP-8.2 and IBMP-8.4), CD signal suggests that these molecules have a post-heating renaturation capacity. Despite denatured, IBMP-8.3 protein did not exhibit aggregate formation as observed by DLS analysis. No significant aggregation was also observed for the IBMP-8.1 and IBMP-8.4 chimeric proteins, although there is an increase in polydispersity for IBMP-8.4. Only IBMP-8.2 presented aggregate formation. Indeed, the hydrodynamic radius substantially changed from 3.7 to 12.5 (Peak 1; %M: 4.7; Pd 12.3), 96.8 (Peak 2; %M: 5.2; Pd 12.3) and 376.3 (Peak 3; %M: 90.17; Pd 18.9). These findings indicate the formation of large protein aggregates, despite monodispersing (Pd < 20). Considering the polyacrylamide gels, no significant degradation was observed with the IBMP proteins. Despite the denaturing conditions, all antigens continue to be recognized by anti-*T. cruzi* antibodies, indicating little of their diagnostic capacity was lost. Indeed, individual epitopes remained available for antigen-antibody interaction.

At 25 °C, all IBMP chimeric proteins proved to be stable for three days (72 h), according to the absence of changes in the CD-spectra. DLS analysis also reveals that, except for IBMP 8-1, there is little change in the aggregation state of the protein samples, indicating high solubility for all proteins. SDS-PAGE, used to assess the integrity of proteins, revealed that IBMP-8.1 and IBMP-8.2 can hold some integrity until 72 h exposure at 25 °C. On the other hand, IBMP-8.3 and IBMP-8.4 suffered severe degradation after 48 h. Despite degradation, CD spectra did not significantly change for IBMP-8.3 and IBMP-8.4 at the 72 h period, suggesting that the CD signal came from short sequences with that of the corresponding full-length sequences. Nevertheless, these proteins showed high resistance to proteolysis. Daily analysis of the short-term assay by ELISA demonstrated that IBMP-8.2 and IBMP-8.3 proteins remain reactive to anti-*T. cruzi* antibodies, even 72 h after the beginning of the analysis. On the other hand, IBMP-8.1 and IBMP-8.4 lost their functionalities to recognize anti-*T. cruzi* antibodies. This is probably due to the degradation of essential epitopes used by these antibodies to bind to IBMP antigens.

Long-term stability analysis at 4 °C revealed that all proteins are stable over one year. We observed that the accuracy values did not change significantly among all eight analysis points for the four antigens. Overall, all absorbed proteins have shown stability over 364 days.

Demonstrating the optimal conditions favoring Ag-Ab kinetics can bring insights into the development of diagnostic tests, regardless of the employed platform. For example, as herein demonstrated, proteins undergo structural changes at different environments, depending on its internal interactions' strength and the characteristics of the protein surface within the solvent/buffer. These changes certainly influence the definition of the parameters that are normally used in biosensors, such as interaction buffer, immobilization time on the electrode surface, dilution ratio, etc., as well as assist in the decision identifying the appropriate buffer for sensitizing a microtiter plate for ELISA, or activating magnetic bead's surface in a microarray assay.

5. Conclusions

In this work, we are demonstrating that when diluted in carbonate buffer the IBMP-8.1 to IBMP-8.4 antigens are very stable, and even after some degradation under temperature effect. Furthermore, absorbed proteins were stable for over one year. The main limitation of this study is the lack of data in the scientific literature to compare our findings. However, we believe that the publication of stability analyses provides relevant information for the utilization of recombinant antigens in immunoassays.

Supplementary Materials: The following are available online at https://www.mdpi.com/article/10.3390/bios11080289/s1, Table S1: Individual data points of reversibility of heat-induced denaturation evaluation; Table S2: Individual data points of storage stability at 25 °C evaluation; Table S3: Individual data points of long-term stability analysis at 4 °C.

Author Contributions: All the authors contributed significantly to work described in this article. P.A.F.C., F.L.N.S. and N.I.T.Z. designed the experimental procedure; P.A.F.C., U.D.O. and F.L.N.S. conducted circular dichroism, dynamic scattering light and SDS-PAGE experiments; L.M.L. and F.L.N.S. conducted ELISA experiments; L.M.L., N.E.M.F., Â.A.O.S., R.T.D., E.F.S. and F.L.N.S. helped with writing the paper and prepared figures; N.I.T.Z. and F.L.N.S. wrote the paper; M.A.K., N.I.T.Z. and F.L.N.S. provided lab space and procured funding for this study. F.L.N.S. supervised the work. All authors have read and agreed to the published version of the manuscript.

Funding: This research was funded by the Gonçalo Moniz Institute, Coordination of Superior Level Staff Improvement-Brazil (CAPES; Code 001), Research Support Foundation of the State of Bahia (FAPESB), Inova Fiocruz/VPPCB (VPPCB-008-FIO-18-2-20), FINEP (01.11.0286.00) and BNDES (11.2.1328.1). Marco A Krieger, Nilson I. T. Zanchin and Fred L. N. Santos are CNPq researches fellow (processes no. 304167/2019-3, 312195/2015-0 and 309263/2020-4, respectively).

Institutional Review Board Statement: The study was conducted according to the guidelines of the Declaration of Helsinki, and approved by the Institutional Review Board (IRB) for Human Research at the Gonçalo Moniz Institute of the Oswaldo Cruz Foundation (IGM-FIOCRUZ), Salvador, Bahia-Brazil (CAAE: 67809417.0.0000.0040).

Informed Consent Statement: Informed consent was obtained from all subjects involved in the study. Written informed consent has been obtained from the patient(s) to publish this paper.

Data Availability Statement: Data is contained within the article or supplementary material.

Acknowledgments: The authors acknowledge the Platform for Protein Purification and Characterization [RPT-15A] of the FIOCRUZ Technical Platform Network.

Conflicts of Interest: The authors declare no conflict of interest. The funders had no role in the design of the study; in the collection, analyses, or interpretation of data; in the writing of the manuscript, or in the decision to publish the results.

References

1. Hotez, P.J.; Dumonteil, E.; Woc-Colburn, L.; Serpa, J.A.; Bezek, S.; Edwards, M.S.; Hallmark, C.J.; Musselwhite, L.W.; Flink, B.J.; Bottazzi, M.E. Chagas disease: "The new HIV/AIDS of the Americas". *PLoS Negl. Trop. Dis.* **2012**, *6*, e1498. [CrossRef] [PubMed]
2. Prata, A. Clinical and epidemiological aspects of Chagas disease. *Lancet Infect. Dis.* **2001**, *1*, 92–100. [CrossRef]
3. Santos, F.L.N.; Souza, W.V.; Barros, M.S.; Nakazawa, M.; Krieger, M.A.; Gomes, Y.M. Chronic Chagas disease diagnosis: A comparative performance of commercial enzyme immunoassay tests. *Am. J. Trop. Med. Hyg.* **2016**, *94*, 1034–1039. [CrossRef]
4. Verani, J.R.; Seitz, A.; Gilman, R.H.; LaFuente, C.; Galdos-Cardenas, G.; Kawai, V.; De Lafuente, E.; Ferrufino, L.; Bowman, N.M.; Pinedo-Cancino, V.; et al. Geographic variation in the sensitivity of recombinant antigen-based rapid tests for chronic *Trypanosoma cruzi* infection. *Am. J. Trop. Med. Hyg.* **2009**, *80*, 410–415. [CrossRef] [PubMed]
5. Martin, D.L.; Marks, M.; Galdos-Cardenas, G.; Gilman, R.H.; Goodhew, B.; Ferrufino, L.; Halperin, A.; Sanchez, G.; Verastegui, M.; Escalante, P.; et al. Regional variation in the correlation of antibody and T-cell responses to *Trypanosoma cruzi*. *Am. J. Trop. Med. Hyg.* **2014**, *90*, 1074–1081. [CrossRef]
6. Zingales, B. *Trypanosoma cruzi* genetic diversity: Something new for something known about Chagas disease manifestations, serodiagnosis and drug sensitivity. *Acta Trop.* **2018**, *184*, 38–52. [CrossRef]
7. Leeflang, M.M.G.; Rutjes, A.W.S.; Reitsma, J.B.; Hooft, L.; Bossuyt, P.M.M. Variation of a test's sensitivity and specificity with disease prevalence. *CMAJ* **2013**, *185*, e537–e544. [CrossRef]
8. Leeflang, M.M.G.; Bossuyt, P.M.M.; Irwig, L. Diagnostic test accuracy may vary with prevalence: Implications for evidence-based diagnosis. *J. Clin. Epidemiol.* **2009**, *62*, 5–12. [CrossRef] [PubMed]
9. World Health Organization. *WHO Consultation on International Biological Reference Preparations for Chagas Diagnostic Tests*; WHO: Geneva, Switzerland, 2007.
10. Santos, F.L.N.; Celedon, P.A.F.; Zanchin, N.I.T.; Brasil, T.A.C.; Foti, L.; Souza, W.V.; Silva, E.D.; Gomes, Y.M.; Krieger, M.A. Performance assessment of four chimeric *Trypanosoma cruzi* antigens based on antigen-antibody detection for diagnosis of chronic Chagas disease. *PLoS ONE* **2016**, *11*, e0161100. [CrossRef]
11. Hoft, D.F.; Kim, K.S.; Otsu, K.; Moser, D.R.; Yost, W.J.; Blumin, J.H.; Donelson, J.E.; Kirchhoff, L.V. *Trypanosoma cruzi* expresses diverse repetitive protein antigens. *Infect. Immun.* **1989**, *57*, 1959–1967. [CrossRef]
12. Camussone, C.; Gonzalez, V.; Belluzo, M.S.; Pujato, N.; Ribone, M.E.; Lagier, C.M.; Marcipar, I.S. Comparison of recombinant *Trypanosoma cruzi* peptide mixtures versus multiepitope chimeric proteins as sensitizing antigens for immunodiagnosis. *Clin. Vaccine Immunol.* **2009**, *16*, 899–905. [CrossRef]
13. Montagnani, F.; Paolis, F.; Beghetto, E.; Gargano, N. Use of recombinant chimeric antigens for the serodiagnosis of *Mycoplasma pneumoniae* infection. *Eur. J. Clin. Microbiol. Infect. Dis.* **2010**, *29*, 1377–1386. [CrossRef]
14. Lu, Y.; Li, Z.; Teng, H.; Xu, H.; Qi, S.; He, J.; Gu, D.; Chen, Q.; Ma, H. Chimeric peptide constructs comprising linear B-cell epitopes: Application to the serodiagnosis of infectious diseases. *Sci. Rep.* **2015**, *5*, 13364. [CrossRef]
15. Beghetto, E.; Spadoni, A.; Bruno, L.; Buffolano, W.; Gargano, N. Chimeric antigens of *Toxoplasma gondii*: Toward standardization of toxoplasmosis serodiagnosis using recombinant products. *J. Clin. Microbiol.* **2006**, *44*, 2133–2140. [CrossRef]
16. Hollingshead, S.; Jongerius, I.; Exley, R.M.; Johnson, S.; Lea, S.M.; Tang, C.M. Structure-based design of chimeric antigens for multivalent protein vaccines. *Nat. Commun.* **2018**, *9*, 1–10. [CrossRef]
17. Nuccitelli, A.; Cozzi, R.; Gourlay, L.J.; Donnarumma, D.; Necchi, F.; Norais, N.; Telford, J.L.; Rappuoli, R.; Bolognesi, M.; Maione, D.; et al. Structure-based approach to rationally design a chimeric protein for an effective vaccine against Group B *Streptococcus* infections. *Proc. Natl. Acad. Sci. USA* **2011**, *108*, 10278–10283. [CrossRef]
18. Leony, L.M.; Freitas, N.E.M.; Del-Rei, R.P.; Carneiro, C.M.; Reis, A.B.; Jansen, A.M.; Xavier, S.C.C.; Gomes, Y.M.; Silva, E.D.; Reis, M.G.; et al. Performance of recombinant chimeric proteins in the serological diagnosis of *Trypanosoma cruzi* infection in dogs. *PLoS Negl. Trop. Dis.* **2019**, *13*, e0007545. [CrossRef] [PubMed]
19. Cordeiro, T.A.R.; Martins, H.R.; Franco, D.L.; Santos, F.L.N.; Celedon, P.A.F.; Cantuária, V.L.; de Lana, M.; Reis, A.B.; Ferreira, L.F. Impedimetric immunosensor for rapid and simultaneous detection of Chagas and visceral leishmaniasis for point of care diagnosis. *Biosens. Bioelectron.* **2020**, *169*, 112573. [CrossRef] [PubMed]
20. Santos, F.L.N.; Celedon, P.A.; Zanchin, N.I.; Souza, W.V.; Silva, E.D.; Foti, L.; Krieger, M.A.; Gomes, Y.M. Accuracy of chimeric proteins in the serological diagnosis of chronic Chagas disease—A Phase II study. *PLoS Negl. Trop. Dis.* **2017**, *11*, e0005433. [CrossRef]
21. Del-Rei, R.P.; Leony, L.M.; Celedon, P.A.F.; Zanchin, N.I.T.; Reis, M.G.; Gomes, Y.D.M.; Schijman, A.G.; Longhi, S.A.; Santos, F.L.N. Detection of anti-*Trypanosoma cruzi* antibodies by chimeric antigens in chronic Chagas disease-individuals from endemic South American countries. *PLoS ONE* **2019**, *14*, e0215623. [CrossRef] [PubMed]
22. Dopico, E.; Del-Rei, R.P.; Espinoza, B.; Ubillos, I.; Zanchin, N.I.T.; Sulleiro, E.; Moure, Z.; Celedon, P.A.F.; Souza, W.V.; Silva, E.D.; et al. Immune reactivity to *Trypanosoma cruzi* chimeric proteins for Chagas disease diagnosis in immigrants living in a non-endemic setting. *BMC Infect Dis.* **2019**, *19*, 1–7. [CrossRef]
23. Laemmli, U.K. Cleavage of structural proteins during the assembly of the head of bacteriophage T4. *Nature* **1970**, *227*, 680–685. [CrossRef] [PubMed]
24. Santos, F.L.N.; Campos, A.C.P.; Amorim, L.D.A.F.; Silva, E.D.; Zanchin, N.I.T.; Celedon, P.A.F.; Del-Rei, R.P.; Krieger, M.A.; Gomes, Y.M. Highly accurate chimeric proteins for the serological diagnosis of chronic Chagas disease: A latent class analysis. *Am. J. Trop. Med. Hyg.* **2018**, *99*, 1174–1179. [CrossRef]

25. Santos, F.L.N.; Celedon, P.A.F.; Zanchin, N.I.T.; Leitolis, A.; Crestani, S.; Foti, L.; Souza, W.V.; Gomes, Y.M.; Krieger, M.A.; de Souza, W.V.; et al. Performance assessment of a *Trypanosoma cruzi* chimeric antigen in multiplex liquid microarray assays. *J. Clin. Microbiol.* **2017**, *55*, 2934–2945. [CrossRef] [PubMed]
26. Silva, E.D.; Silva, Â.A.O.; Santos, E.F.; Leony, L.M.; Freitas, N.E.M.; Daltro, R.T.; Ferreira, A.G.P.; Diniz, R.L.; Bernardo, A.R.; Luquetti, A.O.; et al. Development of a new lateral flow assay based on IBMP-8.1 and IBMP-8.4 chimeric antigens to diagnose Chagas disease. *Biomed Res. Int.* **2020**, *2020*, 1803515. [CrossRef] [PubMed]
27. Daltro, R.T.; Leony, L.M.; Freitas, N.E.M.; Silva, Â.A.O.; Santos, E.F.; Del-Rei, R.P.; Brito, M.E.F.; Brandão-Filho, S.P.; Gomes, Y.M.; Silva, M.S.; et al. Cross-reactivity using chimeric *Trypanosoma cruzi* antigens: Diagnostic performance in settings co-endemic for Chagas disease and American cutaneous or visceral leishmaniasis. *J. Clin. Microbiol.* **2019**, *57*. [CrossRef]
28. Rocha-Gaso, M.I.; Villarreal-Gómez, L.J.; Beyssen, D.; Sarry, F.; Reyna, M.A.; Ibarra-Cerdeña, C.N. Biosensors to diagnose Chagas disease: A brief review. *Sensors* **2017**, *17*, 2629. [CrossRef]
29. Janissen, R.; Sahoo, P.K.; Santos, C.A.; da Silva, A.M.; von Zuben, A.A.G.; Souto, D.E.P.; Costa, A.D.T.; Celedon, P.; Zanchin, N.I.T.; Almeida, D.B.; et al. InP nanowire biosensor with tailored biofunctionalization: Ultrasensitive and highly selective disease biomarker detection. *Nano Lett.* **2017**, *17*, 5938–5949. [CrossRef]

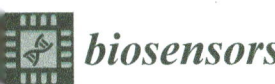

Review

Microfluidic-Chip-Integrated Biosensors for Lung Disease Models

Shuang Ding [1,†], Haijun Zhang [1,*,†] and Xuemei Wang [2,*]

1. Department of Oncology, Zhongda Hospital, School of Medicine, Southeast University, Nanjing 210009, China; dingshuang@seu.edu.cn
2. State Key Laboratory of Bioelectronics, School of Biomedical Engineering, Southeast University, Nanjing 210096, China
* Correspondence: haijunzhang@seu.edu.cn (H.Z.), xuewang@seu.edu.cn (X.W.); Tel.: +86 25 83 792 177 (X.W.)
† These authors contributed equally to this work.

Abstract: Lung diseases (e.g., infection, asthma, cancer, and pulmonary fibrosis) represent serious threats to human health all over the world. Conventional two-dimensional (2D) cell models and animal models cannot mimic the human-specific properties of the lungs. In the past decade, human organ-on-a-chip (OOC) platforms—including lung-on-a-chip (LOC)—have emerged rapidly, with the ability to reproduce the in vivo features of organs or tissues based on their three-dimensional (3D) structures. Furthermore, the integration of biosensors in the chip allows researchers to monitor various parameters related to disease development and drug efficacy. In this review, we illustrate the biosensor-based LOC modeling, further discussing the future challenges as well as perspectives in integrating biosensors in OOC platforms.

Keywords: biosensor; microfluidics; organ-on-a-chip; lung model; lung-on-a-chip

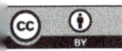

Citation: Ding, S.; Zhang, H.; Wang, X. Microfluidic-Chip-Integrated Biosensors for Lung Disease Models. *Biosensors* **2021**, *11*, 456. https://doi.org/10.3390/bios11110456

Received: 10 October 2021
Accepted: 14 November 2021
Published: 15 November 2021

Publisher's Note: MDPI stays neutral with regard to jurisdictional claims in published maps and institutional affiliations.

Copyright: © 2021 by the authors. Licensee MDPI, Basel, Switzerland. This article is an open access article distributed under the terms and conditions of the Creative Commons Attribution (CC BY) license (https://creativecommons.org/licenses/by/4.0/).

1. Introduction

1.1. Lung Physiology and Diseases

The lungs are among the most important organs in the human body, and are a site for gas exchange. They contain many alveoli with a large total surface area and abundant capillaries wrapped around them. Both alveolar walls and capillary walls are composed of a layer of epithelial cells, which are conducive to gas exchange between the alveoli and the blood. The respiratory membrane is the vital structure for gas exchange, and can be divided into six layers: a liquid layer containing alveolar surfactant, the alveolar epithelial layer, the epithelial basement membrane layer, an interstitial layer between the alveoli and capillaries, the capillary basement membrane layer, and the capillary endothelial cell layer [1]. Common respiratory diseases include inflammation (pneumonia) [2], chronic obstructive pulmonary disease (COPD) [3,4], asthma [5], lung cancer [6–8], pulmonary fibrosis, pulmonary embolism, etc. They occur in different anatomical regions (e.g., alveoli or small airways), with varied pathogenesis and therapeutic principles.

1.2. Microfluidic Chips

In the 1990s, in order to meet the need for more sensitive, efficient, and rapid separation and analysis of biological samples, Manz and Widmer et al. [9] first proposed the concept of miniaturized total analysis systems (μTASs). Today, such systems have developed into one of the most advanced scientific and technological fields in the world. The core technology is based on microfluidic chip systems, or lab-on-a-chip systems [10]. This refers to the integration of sample preparation, reaction, separation, detection, and other basic operational units involved in conventional chemical and biological fields into a chip of several square centimeters, which has the advantages of rapid detection and analysis, large amounts of information, and high throughput. In recent decades, such systems have been widely used in life sciences, disease diagnosis, and drug screening, becoming among the most popular frontier technologies in the 21st century.

1.3. Lung Models

At present, in vitro two-dimensional (2D) cell models/three-dimensional (3D) spheroids, animal models, and human organoid models are commonly used to mimic the lungs, but these models all have their limitations. Monolayer cell culture is simple and cheap, but cannot demonstrate the complex structure and function of the human-organ-specific microenvironment in vivo. 3D spheroids based on hydrogel scaffolds are more similar to the microenvironment, but still have the disadvantages of no perfusion, no stress, and limited vasculature. Animal models, although widely used, are not able to mimic human-specific features, with poor prediction value for patients due to the great differences in respiratory system structure between animal models and humans. Lung organoids can provide a variety of cell types and more complex tissue-specific functions, but they cannot mimic organ-level features of the lungs, such as tissue–tissue interface, epithelial–endothelial crosstalk, and immune cell–host response. These models cannot analyze the recruitment of circulating immune cells under active fluid flow, causing unavoidable problems in the modeling of lung diseases. Therefore, there is an urgent need to develop alternative preclinical models to better mimic the pathophysiology of human lungs. Microfluidic technology is able to handle small volumes of fluids (10^{-9} to 10^{-18} L) across microchannels with dimensions from tens to hundreds of micrometers, which promote the development of human organ-on-a-chip (OOC) systems with the ability to successfully mimic many aspects of the organ-level physiology [11]. A large number of OOC platforms integrated with microfluidic technologies, organ anatomy, physics, materials science, and cell biology have been designed for an array of human organs, including the lungs [12–14], liver [15–17], gut [18,19], kidneys [20,21], and heart [22,23]. Lung-on-a-chip (LOC) [24], as the first proposed OOC, has always been an appealing research topic for mimicking ALI structure or breathing movement, reducing the awkwardness of lung modeling. LOC is a multifunctional microexperimental platform that can reproduce the key structural, functional and mechanical properties of the human alveolar–capillary interface (ACI, the basic functional unit of living lungs), simulate lung function at the organ level, and reflect the tissue–tissue interface, epithelial–endothelial crosstalk, and immune cell–host response. There have been many reports on the application of lung alveolus-on-a-chip and small-airway-on-a-chip systems in simulating lung inflammation, pulmonary edema, pulmonary fibrosis, viral pneumonia, and lung cancer.

1.4. Biosensors

Biosensors are a kind of chemical sensor. They are a signal analysis tool composed of immobilized biologically sensitive material components (including enzymes, antibodies, antigens, microorganisms, cells, tissues, nucleic acids, etc.), corresponding transducers (including oxygen electrodes, photosensitive tubes, field-effect tubes, piezoelectric crystals, etc.), and a signal detecting device. Biosensors [25] are used to detect biological analytes (e.g., biomolecules), structures, and microorganisms, and can monitor and transmit information about a life process [26–28]. As shown in Figure 1, a sensing element (for recognition of biomolecules), signal transducer (for signal translation), and detector (for detecting the signal) make up the sensor. Biosensors were first proposed by Clark et al., who clamped an enzyme solution between two layers of dialysis membrane to form a thin liquid layer, and then glued it to a pH electrode and an oxygen electrode to detect the reaction in the liquid layer. As the lifetime of the enzyme electrode is relatively short, and the purification is also expensive, researchers began to research derivatives of enzyme electrodes—such as animal tissue electrodes, organelle electrodes, and microbial electrodes—which greatly increased the variety of biosensors. According to the sensing principle, the most common integrated sensors can be classified into three groups: electrical [29,30], electrochemical [31–35], and optical [36–38]. Electrical signals are often used to deal with cell growth and responses, while optical and electrochemical sensors are commonly used to detect chemical signals. Various integrated biosensors have been used for chemical analysis in microfluidic chips [39]. The basic concept of the reported microfluidic-based biosensor is to integrate the analysis functions required for biochemical analysis on a single chip, including sample preparation, pretreatment, detection, and molecular sorting. The combination of biosensors and microfluidic chips improves analysis capabilities and broadens the range of possible applications. Recently, some efforts have been made to integrate biosensors into OOC platforms as well.

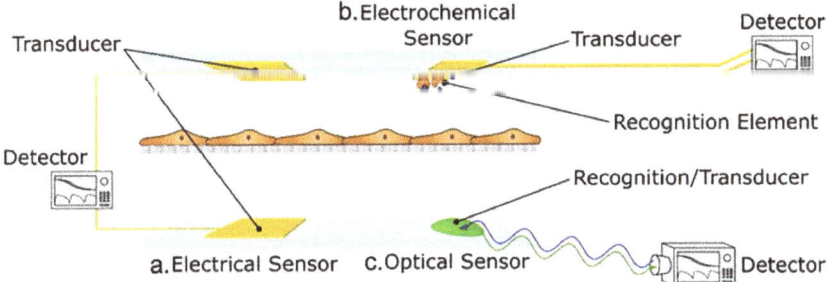

Figure 1. Composition and classification of sensors: Sensors are classified into (a) electrical sensors, (b) electrochemical sensors, and (c) optical sensors. Reproduced with permission from [40].

2. Biosensor-Free LOC for Lung Modeling

The classical "alveolar lung-on-a-chip" [12] and "small airway lung-on-a-chip" [41,42] were established by Huh et al. and Benam et al., respectively, from the Wyss Institute for Biologically Inspired Engineering at Harvard University (Figure 2). In 2010, Huh et al. [12] produced one of the first biomimetic microfluidic lung models, in which 10 μm of polydimethylsiloxane (PDMS) membrane with ECM was sandwiched between the two PDMS microchannels. ALI was generated for gas exchange with the blood. The upper channel contained epithelial cells while the other channel contained microvascular endothelial cells to mimic the ACI. The membrane between the two channels was forced to deform under a vacuum to pneumatic channels on either side of the membrane. The authors found that ALI culture increased the transbilayer electrical resistance (TER, >800 $\Omega \cdot cm^2$) and produced tighter ACI as compared to liquid culture conditions. This study became a pioneer for further studies related to LOCs. Benam et al. [41] introduced a human small airway lung-on-a-chip containing mucociliary bronchiolar epithelium and microvascular endothelium; this chip was made of PDMS containing an upper channel and a parallel lower microvascular channel, which were separated by a polyester membrane coated with type I collagen on both sides. Physiological and pathological processes of the lungs were simulated and developed based on this small airway lung-on-a-chip; the authors also modeled several airway diseases [43,44] (e.g., asthma [45], lung inflammation [42], COPD, and COPD exacerbation [13]) on the chip.

In 2012, Huh et al. mimicked pulmonary edema on a chip [46], the structure of which was similar to the alveolar lung-on-a-chip mentioned above. This pulmonary-edema-on-a-chip reproduced lung function in response to interleukin-2 (IL-2), and also successfully screened a drug for pulmonary edema. Zamprogno et al. [47] presented a second-generation LOC with a lung alveolar array based on a biological, thickness/stiffness-controlled membrane made from collagen and elastin via a simple method. Huang et al. [48] used a model of the human alveoli based on physiological structure; it was composed of a 3D porous hydrogel with an inverse opal structure, and then bonded to a PDMS chip. In contrast to traditional PDMS or biological membranes, the inverse opal hydrogel structure is similar to human alveolar sacs, with well-defined, interconnected pores, and can be introduced to LOCs. Zhang et al. [49,50] evaluated the pulmonary toxicity of TiO_2/ZnO

nanoparticles and fine particulate matter (PM2.5) exposure using a novel three-channel 3D LOC model. Hassell et al. [14] created a chip model of human non-small-cell lung cancer (NSCLC) to recapitulate cancer growth, responses to tyrosine kinase inhibitor (TKI) therapy, and dormancy. Xu et al. [51] reported a multiorgan chip with an upstream "lung" and three downstream "organs", which mimicked the lung cancer metastasis microenvironment. In general, these LOC models mentioned above were biosensor-free, although with different design concepts and applications (see Table 1 for detailed comparisons). Given the biological complexity of the described LOC, future progress must be made in biosensor integration in order to easily monitor related physiological parameters.

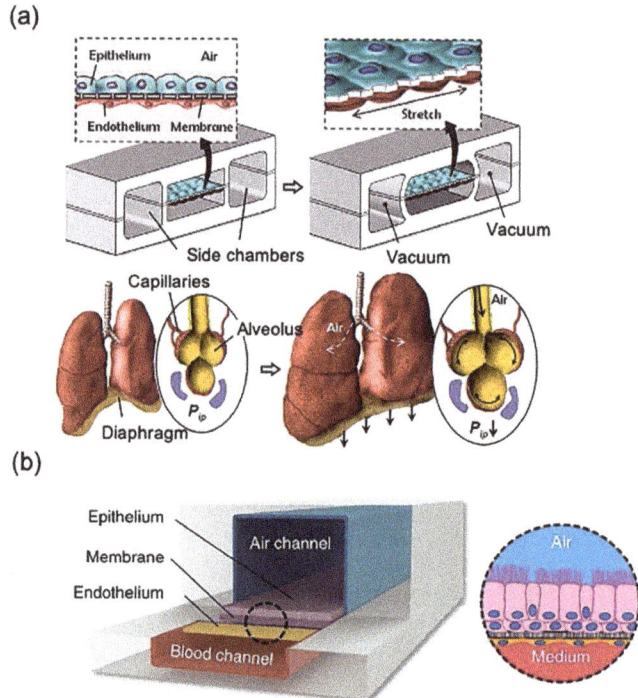

Figure 2. Design of two classical human breathing LOC microdevices: (**a**) Schematic diagram of "alveolar lung-on-a-chip"; physiological breathing movements were reproduced by applying vacuum to the chambers; reproduced with permission from [12]. (**b**) Schematic diagram of the "small airway lung-on-a-chip"; reproduced with permission from [42].

Table 1. Literature review of some biosensor-free LOCs. Chip models, structure of ACI, corresponding remarks, and whether respiration movement was observed are listed in the table for comparison.

Chip Models	Structure of ACI	Remarks	RM [1]	Ref.
Alveolar lung-on-a-chip	Alveolar epithelial cells/PDMS/microvascular endothelium	A pioneer for further studies related to LOC. The authors also introduced pulmonary-edema-on-a-chip to mimic lung function, and screened a new drug for pulmonary edema	Yes	[12]

Table 1. Cont.

Chip Models	Structure of ACI	Remarks	RM [1]	Ref.
Small airway lung-on-a-chip	Differentiated mucociliary bronchiolar epithelium/PDMS/microvascular endothelium	Modeled asthma, lung inflammation, and COPD exacerbation on the chip, and also evaluated the therapeutic response on the chip	With ALI structure	[13,41,42]
A chip model of human NSCLC	Similar to alveolar lung-on-a-chip	Recapitulated cancer growth, responses to TKI therapy, and dormancy	Yes	[14]
Second-generation lung alveolar array	Human primary alveolar epithelial cells (hAEpCs)/collagen–elastin membrane/human lung microvascular endothelial cells	Biological, stretchable, biodegradable, and thickness/stiffness-controlled collagen–elastin membrane outperforms PDMS in many ways.	Yes	[47]
Physiologically relevant model of human alveoli	hAEpCs/alveoli-like 3D GelMA hydrogels/human umbilical vein endothelial cells (results with HUVEC only available in the Supplementary Materials)	3D porous hydrogel with an inverse opal structure bonded to a compartmentalized PDMS chip. Investigated the pathological effects of cigarette smoking and SARS-CoV-2 infection	Yes	[48]
Three-channel 3D LOC model	Alveolar epithelial cells/ECM/pulmonary vascular endothelial cells	Evaluated the pulmonary toxicity of TiO_2/ZnO nanoparticles and PM2.5 exposure	No	[49,50]
Multiorgan lung cancer metastasis-on-a-chip	Human bronchial epithelial and lung cancer cells/PDMS/microvascular endothelial cells, fibroblasts, and macrophages	Upstream "lung" and downstream "brain", "bone", and "liver" to mimic the in vivo microenvironment of cancer metastasis	Yes	[51]

[1] RM refers to respiration movement.

3. Biosensors in Microfluidic Chips for Lung Modeling

Biosensors have been widely used in the field of analysis, as they can carry out online and continuous monitoring in complex systems, with the properties of high automation, miniaturization, and integration. When biosensors are combined with new approaches, they can have a revolutionary impact on biotechnology. In the following section, we mainly introduce microfluidic chips for lung modeling, along with integrated biosensors for detecting related parameters. Although some microfluidic chips do not have the structure of LOCs, they have successfully achieved the sensing of specific parameters, laying a foundation for the integration of biosensors in LOCs.

3.1. Transepithelial Electric Resistance (TEER)

Traditional techniques for the measurement of TEER are not suitable for microfluidic devices that replicate the dynamic microenvironment of lung respiration movements [52]. It is difficult to place the microelectrodes on the chip such that the biomimetic capability of the chip is protected and cells are easily accessed via simple handling.

In 2017, Henry et al. [53] from the Wyss Institute described a newly developed human airway-on-a-chip with embedded electrodes for TEER biosensors (Figure 3). Four electrodes were integrated into a microfluidic device that they developed previously [42]. The chip was fabricated using polycarbonate (PC) as a base substrate for its high optical clarity, cell culture biocompatibility, ease of machining, compatibility with metal deposition processes, and ease of chemical surface modification. Epoxy moieties were introduced at the PDMS surface using GLYMO prior to the binding of plasma-activated PDMS to the silanol groups introduced at the PC surface via aminopropyltriethoxysilane (APTES) treatment. This method improved bonding efficacy and enabled long-term resistance to hydrolytic cleavage. Electrodes were 1 mm wide, spaced 1 mm apart, and patterned on PC substrates using a laser-patterned, silicon-coated, backing paper shadow mask. These electrodes were not only stable, but also transparent, allowing for real-time monitoring using optical microscopy. The authors successfully maintained the chip for 62 days in culture and 56 days at ALI, without any evidence of cell toxicity from the presence of the gold and titanium layers. This biosensor can be used in OOC modelling of barriers (e.g., the blood–brain barrier), as it enables measurement of barrier function in cultured cells.

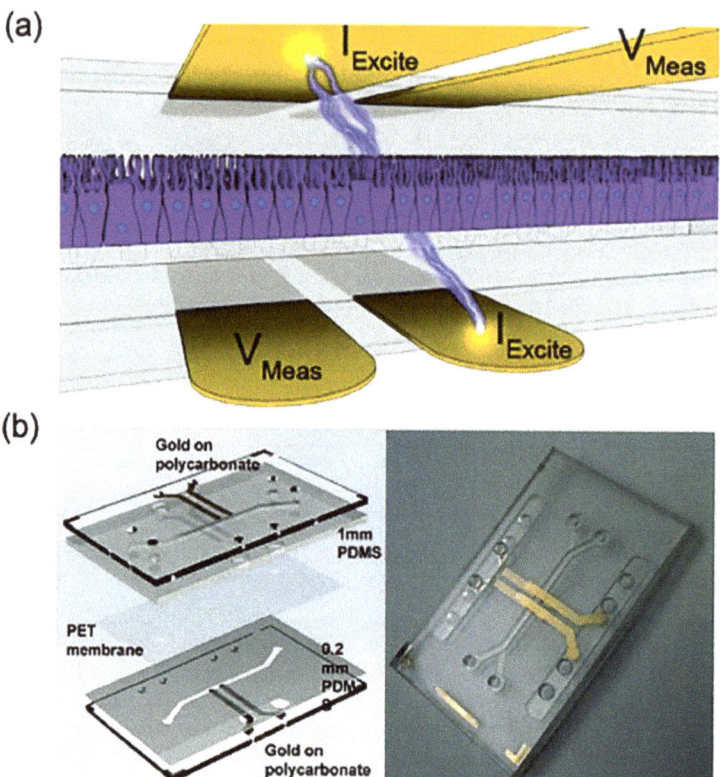

Figure 3. Microengineered human airway-on-a-chip with TEER biosensor: (**a**) Schematic view of the TEER chip's working principle. (**b**) Photograph of the assembled TEER chip. Reproduced with permission from [53].

Increased information output can be obtained by using different types of biosensors in one chip. Khalid et al. [54] introduced a lung-cancer-on-a-chip system equipped with multiple sensors (Figure 4). The chip was prepared in-house by inkjet printing the elastomeric microfluidic channel onto the glass. The top and bottom glasses were held together by a 3D-printed chip holder. During the 54 h real-time monitoring, different concentrations of chemotherapeutics were introduced to NCI-H1437 cells; meanwhile, real-time data of media pH and TEER impedance were obtained via optical pH sensor and top/bottom ITO electrodes. Optical sensors for non-invasive pH monitoring of media were assembled using commercial electronics, white LEDs, optical filters, photodiodes, and 3D printing. The working principle is that when the pH of the extracellular culture medium changes, the color of phenolic red in the culture medium flowing through transparent and biocompatible microfluidic channels changes, and the change in pH can be quantified by measuring the change in light intensity in the channels. Optical pH sensors were characterized and calibrated in the pH range 6.0–8.5 using standard pH media samples. The culture media pH and impedance were monitored for 2 days without any problems in a typical experiment. Then, 500 nm transparent indium tin oxide (ITO)-based TEER impedance-sensing electrodes were patterned using the photolithography technique. The active area of the electrodes was 16 mm^2. The TEER impedance data converted to the cell index (CI) (normalized impedance values) showed that an increase in the drug concentrations caused higher cell death rates. The authors concluded that increased drug concentration caused medium acidification and higher cell death rates due to an increase in the number of acidic molecules; furthermore, these sensors could also be used in drug screening systems, and the chip introduced by the authors was also a promising tool for the development of personalized medicine.

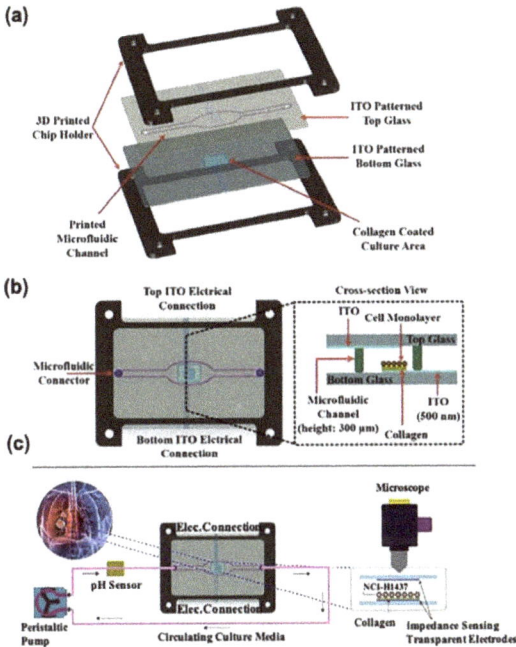

Figure 4. Lung-cancer-on-chip system with multiple sensors: (a) Cross-section view and (b) top view of microfluidic glass chip fabrication. (c) Working flow of the chip for physiological environment monitoring and drug cytotoxicity evaluation. Reproduced with permission from [54].

Mermoud et al. [55] reported a new micro-impedance tomography (MITO) system with the ability to monitor changes in the lung alveolar barrier at a distance of 1 mm from the electrodes using impedimetric coplanar electrodes (Figure 5). They integrated the system into an LOC that models breathing movement through a thin film, based on their previous study [56]. The sensing system was produced using a printed circuit board (PCB). The electrodes on the PCB consisted of 35 μm of copper covered with an electroless nickel plating and a 50 nm thick layer of immersion gold. The flexible PCB was irreversibly bonded with oxygen plasma between the actuation membrane and the actuation part, providing the LOC with barrier function monitoring in a simple, cost-effective manner.

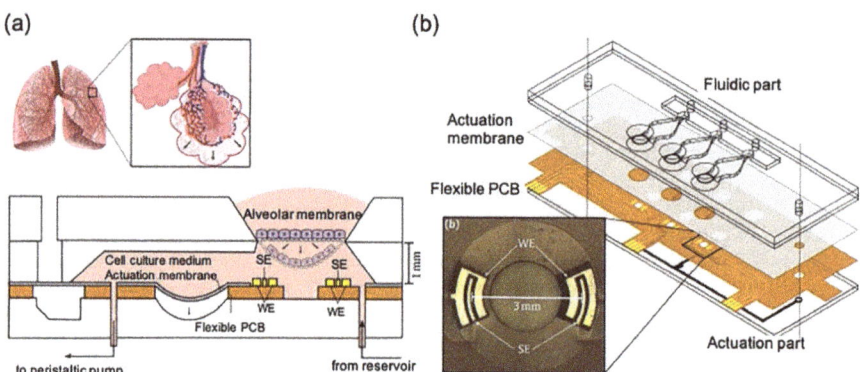

Figure 5. LOC integrated with a MITO system: (**a**) Cross-sectional view of the system. (**b**) Detailed information about the flexible PCB that can be bonded between two layers in the LOC. Reproduced with permission from [55].

The single-organ LOC can mimic lung cell culture microenvironments, but cannot reproduce the interactions between the lungs and other organs. Combining multiple organ types within a single chip can better model the in vivo microenvironment, and is urgently needed. Skardal et al. [57] described a three-tissue OOC system (liver, heart, and lungs; see Figure 6). Liver and cardiac organoids were integrated into a circulatory perfusion system, which was connected to a lung module with an ALI. Lung modules were composed of endothelial cells, lung fibroblasts, and epithelial cells over a semi-permeable membrane within the chip. Transepithelial resistance (TEER) and short-circuit current (Isc) electrophysiological sensing functions were realized by advanced electrodes. The surfaces of the electrodes were functionalized by immobilizing streptavidin (SPV) on the working electrode via covalent bonding with EDC/NHS. The system was maintained for more than 9 days, with direct monitoring of organoid integrity and organ function. The authors found that bleomycin—a drug that causes lung fibrosis and inflammation—also caused toxicity in the cardiac organoids by releasing inflammatory cytokines, including IL-1β. The advanced in vitro drug screening capability of the system represents an important contribution to the field of drug development.

As the most commonly used type of biosensors in OOCs, electrical sensors measure voltage to determine cell properties and physical properties. Optical sensing relies on various forms of microscopy, without consumption of the analyte. Electrochemical sensors work by catalyzing an analyte into another active product. With the application of sensors in biology, more and more biosensors are used to detect biochemical indicators, and not simply to detect some physical parameters. In the following section, we mainly classify the different sensing targets—such as respiratory viruses, biomarkers (e.g., deoxyribonucleic acid (DNA), ribonucleic acid (RNA), proteins, cells), drug efficacy, oxygen, temperature, etc.—in biosensor-based microfluidic chips for lung modeling.

3.2. Respiratory Virus Infections

Since 2019, COVID-19 has been a global pandemic. The current gold standard for diagnosis is viral nucleic acid testing, which is time consuming and labor intensive. Therefore, there is an urgent need for a fast and accurate virus detection method. Qiu et al. [58] reported a dual-functional plasmonic biosensor combining the plasmonic photothermal (PPT) effect and localized surface plasmon resonance (LSPR) to sense transduction for the clinical diagnosis of COVID-19. On the one hand, complementary DNA-receptor-functionalized two-dimensional gold nano-islands (AuNIs) can achieve sensitive detection of the selected sequences from severe acute respiratory syndrome coronavirus 2 (SARS-CoV-2) via nucleic acid hybridization. On the other hand, the AuNIs can enhance the sensing performance by generating thermoplasmonic heat. Jin et al. [59] developed a useful system for the detection of human respiratory adenovirus (HAdV) by combining a biosensor with a microfluidic sample processing module. The detection of viral DNA was accomplished by using a bio-optical sensor of isothermal solid-phase DNA amplification after the DNA was extracted from clinical samples within 30 min using a disposable thin film to facilitate the viral DNA extraction from clinical samples.

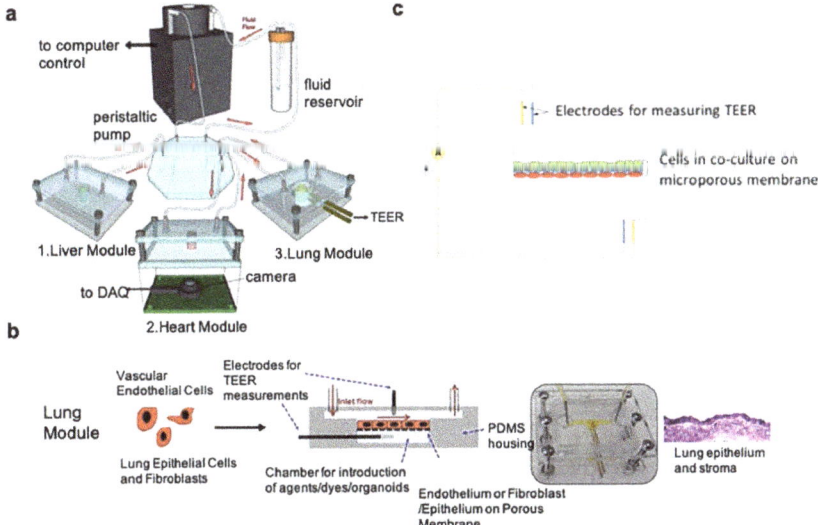

Figure 6. Overall design of the 3-tissue OOC system: (a) Illustration of the system. (b) Lung modules are formed within microfluidic devices. (c) TEER sensors in lung modules are introduced to monitor tissue barrier function over time. Reproduced with permission from [57].

3.3. Lung Cancer Biomarkers

Biomarkers refer to biomolecules that are signs of normal or abnormal processes, conditions, or diseases found in bodily fluids or tissues. They can be used to monitor the progression and efficacy of a disease—especially in cancer [60–65]. Biomarkers include DNA, RNA, and proteins (e.g., antigens, cytokines). They are widely detected in bodily fluids such as blood, urine, saliva, tears, and cerebrospinal fluid. Combined detection of multiple tumor markers can improve the sensitivity and specificity of tumor diagnosis. In the following section, biosensors for lung cancer at the molecular level (DNA, RNA, and proteins), organelle level (exosomes), and cell level (circulating tumor cells (CTCs)) are comprehensively discussed.

3.3.1. Molecular Level (DNA, RNA, and Proteins)

DNA [66,67], RNA [68,69], and proteins play important roles in early-stage cancer diagnosis, but their detection remains a challenge because of low expression levels [70–72]. Traditionally, cancer-related circulating tumor DNA (ctDNA) is usually detected via personalized analysis of rearranged ends (PARE), whole-genome sequencing, or digital PCR-based methods. MicroRNAs (miRNAs) [73], as a class of small, non-coding endogenous RNAs of ~22 nucleotides long, are traditionally detected by real-time qPCR, Northern blotting, microarray, and deep transcriptome sequencing (RNA-Seq). Lung cancer protein biomarkers [74–76]—such as antigens (NSE, SCC, etc.), MMPs, and cytokines—are widely used in clinical practice. Extensive efforts have been devoted to developing ultrasensitive biosensors for the detection of cancer protein biomarkers.

Sheng et al. [77] introduced a dual signal amplification strategy, which was integrated on an electrochemical biosensor for the rapid detection of RNAs (miRNA-17, miRNA-155, miRNA-19b, miRNA-210, thyroid transcription factor-1 messenger RNA (TTF-1 mRNA) and epidermal growth factor receptor (EGFR) mRNA). This platform could selectively and sensitively distinguish early-stage NSCLC patients from healthy controls and benign lung disease patients by identifying low-expression RNA targets in human sera. Portela et al. [78] employed simple colloidal lithography to build a cm^2-sized nanostructured plasmonic biosensor chip based on nanogap antennas. miRNA-210, a biomarker of lung cancer, was detected by this chip via a DNA/miRNA hybridization assay. The sensing potential was proven to be excellent, owing to a limit of detection (LOD) of 0.78 nM. Aoki et al. [79] fabricated a 384-channel biosensor array chip for the detection of multiple mRNAs and miRNAs for lung cancer. The individual biosensor was composed of a photolithographically fabricated Au/Cr-based electrode modified with peptide nucleic acid (PNA) probes. Sequence-specific responses were proven on the chip with an LOD of 73.3 nM. Furthermore, potential use with polymerase chain reaction (PCR) samples was suggested by PCR-amplified oligonucleotide samples. Zeng et al. [80] developed a novel anchor-like DNA (alDNA) electrochemical biosensor for the detection of Kirsten rat sarcoma viral oncogene (KRAS) point mutation level. Compared to the conventional ligation-based DNA biosensors, the alDNA biosensor was convenient and cheap, with high sensitivity and selectivity; it could capture both wild-type and mutant DNA in one step. Furthermore, mutation detection in blood samples could meet the requirements for early-stage NSCLC diagnosis in clinical settings. Wu et al. [81] developed a chip consisting of gold-coated cover glass and tethered cationic lipoplex nanoparticles (tCLN) containing molecular beacons (MBs), which could capture cancer-cell-derived exosomes or viruses and identify encapsulated RNAs in a single step. The CLNs were able to fuse with the exosomes and form nanoparticle complexes via electrostatic interaction. Then, the MBs hybridized with the target RNAs, and exosomes enriched in the target RNAs were detected by the fluorescence signals of MBs using total internal reflection fluorescence (TIRF) microscopy. Furthermore, only 60 µL of serum and 2.5 h were needed in this system, which showed very promising prospects in the detection of exo-miRNAs and clinical diagnosis.

Chiu et al. [82] constructed a signal amplification sensing film for the detection of the cytokeratin 19 fragment (CYFRA21-1). This novel surface plasmon resonance (SPR) detection assay was ultrasensitive, with an LOD of 0.05 pg/mL in spiked clinical sera, which is 10^4 times more sensitive than an enzyme-linked immunosorbent assay (ELISA). Cheng et al. [83] developed field-effect transistor (FET) biosensors to detect CYFRA21-1 and neuron-specific enolase (NSE) in both serum and phosphate-buffered saline (PBS); they also integrated two antibody types on the same chip for simultaneous multiplexed detection. Zou et al. [84] introduced a chip cartridge packaged with a Love wave biosensor for the measurement of CEA, NSE, and squamous-cell carcinoma (SCC) antigen in exhaled breath condensate (EBC) collected from both healthy volunteers and lung cancer patients; gold nanoparticles were immobilized onto the biosensor by a sandwich immunoassay. In addition to tumor markers, specific antigens involved in different processes of disease can also help in the diagnosis and prognosis of disease, such as epithelial–mesenchymal transition (EMT) transcription factor, and inflammatory indicators such as C-reactive protein (CRP) and procalcitonin (PCT). Chakravarty et al. [85] demonstrated a silicon chip platform integrated with photonic crystal (PC) microcavity biosensors to detect the EMT transcription factor zinc finger E-box-binding homeobox 1 (ZEB1) in lysates from NCI-H358 cells. The shift in resonance wavelength resulting from the changed refractive index in the PC microcavity could detect the binding of the corresponding antigen. Feng et al. [86] integrated a microelectrode and a cathodic photoelectrochemical (PEC) biosensor into a microfluidic chip for the detection of CYFRA21-1, based on a signal amplification strategy with a detection limit of 0.026 pg/mL.

In addition to the detection of individual biomarkers, multivariate detection has also been widely practiced. Washburn et al. [87] described the simultaneous detection of eight cancer biomarkers (alpha fetoprotein (AFP), activated leukocyte cell adhesion molecule (ALCAM), cancer antigen 15-3 (CA15-3), cancer antigen 19-9 (CA19-9), cancer antigen 125 (CA-125), carcinoembryonic antigen (CEA), osteopontin, and prostate-specific antigen

(PSA)) in serum using an antibody-based sandwich assay, in 1 h, based on silicon photonic biosensors. Gao et al. [88] designed a giant magnetoresistance (GMR) multi-biomarker immunoassay biosensor that could simultaneously detect 12 kinds of tumor marker (AFP, CEA, CYFRA21-1, NSE, SCC, PG I, PG II, CA19-9, total PSA, free PSA, free-beta-hCG, and Tg) to screen patients with lung cancer, liver cancer, digestive tract cancer, prostate cancer, etc. The GMR sensor chip was based on a double-antibody sandwich immunoassay method. Gao et al. [89] developed a label-free assay for the multiplexed detection of lung cancer biomarkers (miRNA-126 and CEA) using silicon nanowire field-effect transistor (SiNW-FET) sensors. Integration of the SiNW sensor and PDMS microfluidic device enables rapid, sensitive, and multiplexed detection.

3.3.2. Organelle Level (Exosomes)

Cancer-derived exosomes [90–92] with a size of 30-150 nm and density of 1.13–1.19 g/mL have drawn much attention in recent decades, and can be obtained from bodily fluids (such as serum, plasma, or urine). They carry a variety of information on the tumor and tumor microenvironment; thus, they play important roles in tumorigenesis and progression. The detection of such biomarkers is useful for the early diagnosis and drug sensitivity analysis of cancer. Yang et al. [93] presented a novel microfluidic device for the isolation and in situ detection of lung-cancer-specific exosomes collected from patients' urine. The integrated biosensor was fabricated using poly(methyl methacrylate) (PMMA) and a nonporous gold (Au) nanocluster membrane modified with the capture antibody. The change in scattering intensity due to resonance Rayleigh scattering enables the ultrasensitive detection of exosomes.

3.3.3. Cell Level (Circulating Tumor Cells (CTCs))

CTCs are the tumor cells that are separated from the primary solid tumor and enter the bloodstream for various reasons. They play an important role in early diagnosis, detection of tumor recurrence and metastasis, prognostic evaluation, and treatment guidance. The detection and characterization of CTCs provide a non-invasive approach for monitoring cancer therapy. Chen et al. [94] designed a magnet-deformability hybrid integrated microfluidic chip to enumerate CTCs. NSCLC patient blood samples were used to validate the microfluidic chip clinically, with a high capture efficiency (over 90% at 3 mL/h) and high viability (96%) at high flow rates. Nguyen et al. [95] combined dielectrophoretic (DEP) manipulation and impedance measurement using a single microfluidic device equipped with circular microelectrodes to detect CTCs; the force of DEP and hydrodynamic drag drove A549 lung cancer cells to the center of the working region; the LOD of the impedance biosensor was approximately three cells. The same group [96] also introduced a microdevice with electrical sensors based on aptamer-modified gold electrodes for the detection of A549 cells. This device permitted not only optical microscope observations, but also electrical impedance spectroscopy (EIS) measurements. Nabovati et al. [97] introduced an array of charge-based capacitive measurement biosensors for high-throughput cell growth monitoring; the authors tested both H1299 cells and polystyrene beads, with consistent results with cell-based assays; the results showed that the capacitive electrodes can successfully detect cell attachment and growth. Do et al. [98] combined a DEP microfluidic enrichment platform with a capacitive biosensor to detect CTCs; A549 cells were driven to the working chamber via DEP forces, and then captured by an anti-EGFR modified electrode; finally, cells were detected according to their different capacitance. Li et al. [99] developed a cell isolation microfluidic device based on electrotactic ability; this chip was composed of three parts: a cell immobilization structure, an electric field (EF) generator, and a cell retrieval module. The results show that H1975 cell motility was related to EGFR expression and upregulation of ras homolog family member A (RhoA), regardless of EF stimulation, while it was also related to phosphatase and tensin homolog deleted on chromosome ten (PTEN) expression in the presence of EF stimulation.

3.4. Drug Efficacy

Drug efficacy evaluation is important in clinical treatment and drug development. Traditionally, the measurement of cell responses to drugs requires cell counting kit-8 (CCK8), methyl thiazolyl tetrazolium (MTT) assays, animal models, etc., but the biosensor-equipped chip simplifies this process. The corresponding result can be read directly through the biosensor. Pan et al. [100] developed a microgroove impedance sensor (MGIS) for monitoring 3D A549 cell viability in a dynamic and non-invasive manner. Cells were planted in microgrooves for in situ impedance measurement. The proliferation and apoptosis of cells indicated by the change in the living cell number caused an inversely proportional change in the impedance magnitude. The results based on this MGIS platform were very similar to the clinically observed effects of chemotherapy on NSCLC. Noh et al. [101] reported in-air monitoring of in vitro monolayer cells by EIS; two chambers in the chip were separated by a porous membrane, on which EIS electrodes were patterned and A549 cells were cultured. Unlike conventional TEER, electrodes were placed laterally—instead of vertically—to the membrane. This in-air EIS biosensor can enable not only the monitoring of cell population, but also the modulation of tight junctions.

3.5. Oxygen and Temperature

Oxygen and temperature are two of the most important physical parameters in the process of cell culture. Although important, they are the most easily ignored parameters, because of the difficulty in simply reading out these indicators in the traditional culture process. Zirath et al. [102] developed two microfluidic devices integrated with oxygen-sensitive, microparticle-based biosensor spots. The microdevice was composed of two glass substrates, onto which sensor microparticles were pipetted directly; an adhesive film containing the fluidic structure bonded the two layers together. Partial oxygen pressures, cellular oxygen consumption rates with varying cell types, flow rates, and cell numbers were monitored.

Temperature changes in cells are closely connected with physiological processes. Temperature measurements are beneficial to the study of cellular mechanisms. Zhao et al. [103] developed a microfluidic chip for cellular temperature monitoring using a platinum (Pt) thermosensor. The chip was positioned in a constant water tank 24 h after cell seeding. The results showed that temperature response to cisplatin differed in different cells. In conclusion, this chip could be applied to study cell physiology and pathology, with the ability to monitor cellular temperature.

In general, microfluidic chips integrated with biosensors for lung disease modeling, with different design concepts and applications, are briefly summarized in Table 2.

Table 2. Literature review of some biosensor-based microfluidic chips for lung disease modeling. Detailed sensing parameters and characteristics of corresponding sensing technology are listed for summary.

Sensing Parameter	Sample	Keywords	Advantages	Ref.
Respiratory virus	SARS-CoV-2	A dual-functional plasmonic biosensor combining the plasmonic photothermal (PPT) effect and localized surface plasmon resonance (LSPR) for sensing transduction	High sensitivity; lower detection limit; cost-effective	[58]
	HAdV	Bio-optical sensor of isothermal solid-phase DNA amplification; a disposable thin film to facilitate the extraction of viral DNA	Low-cost; simplicity; fast (30 min); simple instruments	[59]

Table 2. Cont.

Sensing Parameter	Sample	Keywords	Advantages	Ref.
DNA/RNA biomarkers	miR-17, miR-155, TTF1mRNA, miR-19b, miR-210	CRISPR/CHDC system; early cancer diagnosis	High sensitivity; low-cost; easy scalability; short assay time	[77]
	miR-210	Large-area nano-plasmonic biosensor; nanogap antennas; customized colloidal lithography process	Simple; low-cost; direct and label-free detection; high sensitivity	[78]
	IGFBP5, EGR3, TFF1 mRNAs, miR-17, miR-21, miR-223	384-Channel, photolithographically fabricated electrode; Au/Cr-based; PNA probes modified	Simple; low cost; simultaneous detection	[79]
	KRAS point mutation	alDNA electrochemical biosensor	High accuracy; convenient, low-cost, and time-saving, with broad dynamic range, and high sensitivity and selectivity	[80]
	miR-21 and TTF-1 mRNA	Tethered cationic lipoplex nanoparticles (tCLN) containing molecular beacons (MBs),	Non-invasive and highly sensitive	[81]
Protein biomarkers	CYFRA21-1	Carboxyl-functionalized molybdenum disulfide (carboxyl-MoS2) nanocomposites; signal amplification sensing film	High specificity	[82]
	CYFRA21-1, NSE	FET biosensor	Simple and rapid; low sample consumption; cheap	[83]
	CEA, NSE and SCC	Tumor markers; clinical EBC samples; gold nanoparticle sandwich immunoassay	Sensitive, specific, and rapid; low cost of time and money; low sample volume	[84]
	ZEB1 in lysates from NCI-H358 cells	Photonic crystal (PC) microcavity biosensors	Duplicate or triplicate analyses; high sensitivity and specificity	[85]
	CYFRA21-1	A microelectrode and a cathodic photoelectrochemical (PEC) biosensor based on a signal amplification strategy	Rapid detection; high selectivity; cost-effectiveness	[86]
	AFP, ALCAM, CA15-3, CA19-9, CA-125, CEA, Osteopontin, PSA	Eight cancer biomarkers in serum; antibody-based sandwich assay	Rapid (1 h) and fully automated	[87]
	AFP, CEA, CYFRA21-1, NSE, SCC, PG I, PG II, CA19-9, total PSA, free PSA, free-beta-hCG, Tg	A giant magnetoresistance (GMR) multi-biomarker immunoassay biosensor; simultaneously detects 12 kinds of tumor markers	High throughput; excellent sensitivity, accuracy, precision, and stability; convenient	[88]

Table 2. Cont.

Sensing Parameter	Sample	Keywords	Advantages	Ref.
	miRNA-126 and CEA	Silicon nanowire field-effect transistor (SiNW-FET)	Multiplexed real-time monitoring; high sensitivity and selectivity; label-free; low-cost	[89]
Exosomes	Lung-cancer-specific exosomes	Isolation and in situ detection; collected from patients' urine; nanoporous gold (Au) nanocluster membrane modified with the capture antibody	Fast and ultrasensitive; simultaneous isolation and detection	[93]
CTCs/rare cells	CTCs from NSCLC patient blood	A magnet-deformability hybrid integrated microfluidic chip, validated clinically with a high capture efficiency	Versatile and high-efficiency; size/deformability hybrid	[94]
	A549	DEP manipulation; impedance measurement; circular microelectrodes	Simple; rapid; label-free; low-cost	[95]
	A549	Amine-terminated aptamer-modified gold electrodes; early-stage lung cancer	Simple; cheap; biocompatible	[96]
	H1299 cells	An array of charge-based capacitive measurement biosensors for high-throughput cell growth monitoring	Label-free and real-time detection; high throughput; high sensitivity	[97]
	A549	Guided and captured; electrode immobilized by anti-EGFR	High sensitivity	[98]
	H1975 cell	Composed of cell immobilization structure, electric field (EF) generator, and cell retrieval module	Easy cell manipulation and precise field control	[99]
Drug efficacy	A549	MGIS; dynamic and noninvasive monitoring; 3D cell viability	Real-time; noninvasive; high throughput	[100]
	A549	EIS; in-air monitoring	In situ and real-time monitoring of "air-exposed" cells	[101]
Oxygen	A549, HUVEC, ASC, NHDF	Oxygen-sensitive microparticle-based biosensor spot arrays	Non-invasive, real-time, label-free in situ monitoring of oxygen demands and metabolic activity	[102]
Temperature	H1975	Pt thermosensor; cellular temperature monitoring	Non-disposable and label-free	[103]

4. Conclusions and Future Perspectives

Biosensors are a new technology developed by combining biotechnology and electronic technology. They have the advantages of good selectivity, high sensitivity, fast analysis speed, and low cost, and can carry out continuous online monitoring in complex systems. Biosensors also have the advantages of high automation, miniaturization, and integration, which greatly reduce the requirements for the working environment. They are very suitable for field analysis, and have important application value in the fields of biology, medicine, environmental monitoring, food, medicine, and military medicine. The development of biosensors has generally gone through the following three stages: (1) the first generation of biosensors consists of electrochemical electrodes and inactive matrix membranes (dialysis membranes or reaction membranes) with fixed biological components; (2) the second generation of biosensors—biological components directly adsorbed or covalently bound to the surface of the converter—do not need the inactive matrix membrane, and do not need to add other reagents to the sample; (3) in the third generation of biosensors, biological components are directly fixed on the electronic components, and can directly sense and amplify the changes in interface substances, so as to combine biometric recognition and signal conversion processing. Biosensors have been incorporated into OOC platforms for a long time, in order to allow for in situ, real-time, small-volume detection of biochemical parameters with minor disturbances to the system [29,37,104–110]. In this review, we summarized biosensor-free (Table 1) and biosensor-integrated (Table 2) LOC models, illustrating the chip design and sensing signals of biosensor-integrated LOCs in detail by using examples of related studies. Biosensor research requires interdisciplinary knowledge of microfabrication, microengineering, materials science, chemistry, and biology. Major challenges for the successful integration of biosensors into OOC platforms are their miniaturization [111], biocompatibility, and flexibility. The trends in this field are as follows: (a) integrating more than one biosensor type, allowing for increased information acquisition and an increased feasibility of the model; and (b) increasing the detection ability of precise and personalized clinical testing devices. In summary, microfluidic-based biosensors play an important role in achieving high-throughput, highly sensitive, low-cost analysis. There is still a long way to go in the further development of integrated biosensors in LOCs, until more biosensors are explored and the advantages compared to off-chip assays are fully appreciated. Hopefully, this review will help both biologists and engineers to turn their minds to further development in the integration of biosensors in LOCs. The integration of microfluidic chips and biosensors has overcome the main difficulties in the initial stage of development, such as processing technology and flow control technology. The field is moving into a transformative period, where deeper basic research, extensive application, and in-depth industrialization should be accomplished. It is expected that in the near future, the sensor detection systems in microfluidic chips will replace complex equipment in traditional chemical analysis laboratories, and "personalized laboratories" that can monitor disease-related biochemical indicators will become a reality.

Author Contributions: Conceptualization, X.W. and H.Z.; writing—original draft preparation, S.D.; writing—review and editing, H.Z.; supervision, X.W. All authors have read and agreed to the published version of the manuscript.

Funding: This research was funded by the Fundamental Research Funds for the Central Universities and the Ordinary University Graduate Student Research Innovation Project of Jiangsu Province, China (KYCX18_0185), and the Science and Technology Grants of Jiangsu Province (BE2019716 and BE2019738).

Institutional Review Board Statement: Not applicable.

Informed Consent Statement: Not applicable.

Data Availability Statement: Not applicable.

Conflicts of Interest: The authors declare no conflict of interest.

References

1. Haefeli-Bleuer, B.; Weibel, E.R. Morphometry of the human pulmonary acinus. *Anat. Rec.* **1988**, *220*, 401–414. [CrossRef]
2. Mandell, L.A.; Niederman, M.S. Aspiration Pneumonia. *N. Engl. J. Med.* **2019**, *380*, 651–663. [CrossRef]
3. Lopez-Campos, J.L.; Tan, W.; Soriano, J.B. Global burden of COPD. *Respirology* **2016**, *21*, 14–23. [CrossRef]

4. Singh, D.; Agusti, A.; Anzueto, A.; Barnes, P.J.; Bourbeau, J.; Celli, B.R.; Criner, G.J.; Frith, P.; Halpin, D.M.G.; Han, M.; et al. Global Strategy for the Diagnosis, Management, and Prevention of Chronic Obstructive Lung Disease: The GOLD science committee report 2019. *Eur. Respir. J.* **2019**, *53*, 1900164. [CrossRef]
5. Papi, A.; Brightling, C.; Pedersen, S.E.; Reddel, H.K. Asthma. *Lancet* **2018**, *391*, 783–800. [CrossRef]
6. Lemjabbar-Alaoui, H.; Hassan, O.U.; Yang, Y.W.; Buchanan, P. Lung cancer: Biology and treatment options. *Biochim. Biophys. Acta (BBA) Bioenerg.* **2015**, *1856*, 189–210. [CrossRef] [PubMed]
7. Barta, J.A.; Powell, C.A.; Wisnivesky, J.P. Global Epidemiology of Lung Cancer. *Ann. Glob. Health* **2019**, *85*. [CrossRef] [PubMed]
8. Siegel, R.L.; Miller, K.D.; Fuchs, H.E.; Jemal, A. Cancer Statistics, 2021. *CA Cancer J. Clin.* **2021**, *71*, 7–33. [CrossRef]
9. Harrison, D.J.; Manz, A.; Fan, Z.H.; Ludi, H.; Widmer, H.M. Capillary electrophoresis and sample injection systems integrated on a planar glass chip. *Anal. Chem.* **1992**, *64*, 1926–1932. [CrossRef]
10. Thorsen, T.; Maerkl, S.J.; Quake, S.R. Microfluidic large-scale integration. *Science* **2002**, *298*, 580–584. [CrossRef]
11. Bhatia, S.N.; Ingber, D.E. Microfluidic organs-on-chips. *Nat. Biotechnol.* **2014**, *32*, 760–772. [CrossRef]
12. Huh, D.; Matthews, B.D.; Mammoto, A.; Montoya-Zavala, M.; Hsin, H.Y.; Ingber, D.E. Reconstituting organ-level lung functions on a chip. *Science* **2010**, *328*, 1662–1668. [CrossRef]
13. Benam, K.H.; Novak, R.; Nawroth, J.; Hirano-Kobayashi, M.; Ferrante, T.C.; Choe, Y.; Prantil-Baun, R.; Weaver, J.C.; Bahinski, A.; Parker, K.K.; et al. Matched-Comparative Modeling of Normal and Diseased Human Airway Responses Using a Microengineered Breathing Lung Chip. *Cell Syst.* **2016**, *3*, 456–466.e4. [CrossRef]
14. Hassell, B.A.; Goyal, G.; Lee, E.; Sontheimer-Phelps, A.; Levy, O.; Chen, C.S.; Ingber, D.E. Human Organ Chip Models Recapitulate Orthotopic Lung Cancer Growth, Therapeutic Responses, and Tumor Dormancy In Vitro. *Cell Rep.* **2017**, *21*, 508–516. [CrossRef]
15. Khazali, A.S.; Clark, A.M.; Wells, A. A Pathway to Personalizing Therapy for Metastases Using Liver-on-a-Chip Platforms. *Stem Cell Rev. Rep.* **2017**, *13*, 364–380. [CrossRef]
16. Beckwitt, C.H.; Clark, A.M.; Wheeler, S.; Taylor, D.L.; Stolz, D.B.; Griffith, L.; Wells, A. Liver 'organ on a chip'. *Exp. Cell Res.* **2018**, *363*, 15–25. [CrossRef] [PubMed]
17. Lasli, S.; Kim, H.J.; Lee, K.; Suurmond, C.E.; Goudie, M.; Bandaru, P.; Sun, W.; Zhang, S.; Zhang, N.; Ahadian, S.; et al. A Human Liver-on-a-Chip Platform for Modeling Nonalcoholic Fatty Liver Disease. *Adv. Biosyst.* **2019**, *3*, e1900104. [CrossRef] [PubMed]
18. Ashammakhi, N.; Nasiri, R.; Barros, N.R.; Tebon, P.; Thakor, J.; Goudie, M.; Shamloo, A.; Martin, M.G.; Khademhosseini, A. Gut-on-a-chip: Current progress and future opportunities. *Biomaterials* **2020**, *255*, 120196. [CrossRef]
19. Poceviciute, R.; Ismagilov, R.F. Human-gut-microbiome on a chip. *Nat. Biomed. Eng.* **2019**, *3*, 500–501. [CrossRef] [PubMed]
20. Lee, J.; Kim, S. Kidney-on-a-Chip: A New Technology for Predicting Drug Efficacy, Interactions, and Drug-induced Nephrotoxicity. *Curr. Drug Metab.* **2018**, *19*, 577–583. [CrossRef] [PubMed]
21. Wilmer, M.J.; Ng, C.P.; Lanz, H.L.; Vulto, P.; Suter-Dick, L.; Masereeuw, R. Kidney-on-a-Chip Technology for Drug-Induced Nephrotoxicity Screening. *Trends Biotechnol.* **2016**, *34*, 156–170. [CrossRef] [PubMed]
22. Zhang, Y.S.; Arneri, A.; Bersini, S.; Shin, S.R.; Zhu, K.; Goli-Malekabadi, Z.; Aleman, J.; Colosi, C.; Busignani, F.; Dell'Erba, V.; et al. Bioprinting 3D microfibrous scaffolds for engineering endothelialized myocardium and heart-on-a-chip. *Biomaterials* **2016**, *110*, 45–59. [CrossRef]
23. Sakamiya, M.; Fang, Y.; Mo, X.; Shen, J.; Zhang, T. A heart-on-a-chip platform for online monitoring of contractile behavior via digital image processing and piezoelectric sensing technique. *Med. Eng. Phys.* **2020**, *75*, 36–44. [CrossRef]
24. Potkay, J.A. The promise of microfluidic artificial lungs. *Lab Chip* **2014**, *14*, 4122–4138. [CrossRef]
25. Alhadrami, H.A. Biosensors: Classifications, medical applications, and future prospective. *Biotechnol. Appl. Biochem.* **2018**, *65*, 497–508. [CrossRef] [PubMed]
26. Li, Y.-C.E.; Lee, I.C. The Current Trends of Biosensors in Tissue Engineering. *Biosensors* **2020**, *10*, 88. [CrossRef]
27. Alsabbagh, K.; Hornung, T.; Voigt, A.; Sadir, S.; Rajabi, T.; Lange, K. Microfluidic Impedance Biosensor Chips Using Sensing Layers Based on DNA-Based Self-Assembled Monolayers for Label-Free Detection of Proteins. *Biosensors* **2021**, *11*, 80. [CrossRef]
28. Chao, L.; Shi, H.; Nie, K.; Dong, B.; Ding, J.; Long, M.; Liu, Z. Applications of Field Effect Transistor Biosensors Integrated in Microfluidic Chips. *Nanosci. Nanotechnol. Lett.* **2020**, *12*, 427–445. [CrossRef]
29. Liao, Z.; Wang, J.; Zhang, P.; Zhang, Y.; Miao, Y.; Gao, S.; Deng, Y.; Geng, L. Recent advances in microfluidic chip integrated electronic biosensors for multiplexed detection. *Biosens. Bioelectron.* **2018**, *121*, 272–280. [CrossRef]
30. Sun, T.; Tsuda, S.; Zauner, K.P.; Morgan, H. On-chip electrical impedance tomography for imaging biological cells. *Biosens. Bioelectron.* **2010**, *25*, 1109–1115. [CrossRef]
31. Wang, J.; Wu, C.; Hu, N.; Zhou, J.; Du, L.; Wang, P. Microfabricated electrochemical cell-based biosensors for analysis of living cells in vitro. *Biosensors* **2012**, *2*, 127–170. [CrossRef]
32. Cui, F.; Zhou, Z.; Zhou, H.S. Review-Measurement and Analysis of Cancer Biomarkers Based on Electrochemical Biosensors. *J. Electrochem. Soc.* **2019**, *167*. [CrossRef]
33. Kaur, G.; Tomar, M.; Gupta, V. Development of a microfluidic electrochemical biosensor: Prospect for point-of-care cholesterol monitoring. *Sens. Actuators B Chem.* **2018**, *261*, 460–466. [CrossRef]
34. Kasturi, S.; Torati, S.R.; Eom, Y.; Kim, C. Microvalve-controlled miniaturized electrochemical lab-on-a-chip based biosensor for the detection of beta-amyloid biomarker. *J. Ind. Eng. Chem.* **2021**, *97*, 349–355. [CrossRef]
35. An, L.; Wang, G.; Han, Y.; Li, T.; Jin, P.; Liu, S. Electrochemical biosensor for cancer cell detection based on a surface 3D micro-array. *Lab Chip* **2018**, *18*, 335–342. [CrossRef]

36. Pires, N.M.M.; Dong, T.; Hanke, U.; Hoivik, N. Recent Developments in Optical Detection Technologies in Lab-on-a-Chip Devices for Biosensing Applications. *Sensors* **2014**, *14*, 15458–15479. [CrossRef] [PubMed]
37. Liao, Z.; Zhang, Y.; Li, Y.; Miao, Y.; Gao, S.; Lin, F.; Deng, Y.; Geng, L. Microfluidic chip coupled with optical biosensors for simultaneous detection of multiple analytes: A review. *Biosens. Bioelectron.* **2019**, *126*, 697–706. [CrossRef]
38. Chen, Y.-T.; Lee, Y.-C.; Lai, Y.-H.; Lim, J.-C.; Huang, N.-T.; Lin, C.-T.; Huang, J.-J. Review of Integrated Optical Biosensors for Point-of-Care Applications. *Biosensors* **2020**, *10*, 209. [CrossRef]
39. Xing, Y.; Zhao, L.; Cheng, Z.; Lv, C.; Yu, F.; Yu, F. Microfluidics-Based Sensing of Biospecies. *ACS Appl. Bio Mater.* **2021**, *4*, 2160–2191. [CrossRef]
40. Fuchs, S.; Johansson, S.; Tjell, A.O.; Werr, G.; Mayr, T.; Tenje, M. In-Line Analysis of Organ-on-Chip Systems with Sensors: Integration, Fabrication, Challenges, and Potential. *ACS Biomater. Sci. Eng.* **2021**, *7*, 2926–2948. [CrossRef]
41. Benam, K.H.; Mazur, M.; Choe, Y.; Ferrante, T.C.; Novak, R.; Ingber, D.E. Human Lung Small Airway-on-a-Chip Protocol. *Methods Mol. Biol.* **2017**, *1612*, 345–365. [CrossRef] [PubMed]
42. Benam, K.H.; Villenave, R.; Lucchesi, C.; Varone, A.; Hubeau, C.; Lee, H.H.; Alves, S.E.; Salmon, M.; Ferrante, T.C.; Weaver, J.C.; et al. Small airway-on-a-chip enables analysis of human lung inflammation and drug responses in vitro. *Nat. Methods* **2016**, *13*, 151–157. [CrossRef]
43. Humayun, M.; Chow, C.-W.; Young, E.W.K. Microfluidic lung airway-on-a-chip with arrayable suspended gels for studying epithelial and smooth muscle cell interactions. *Lab Chip* **2018**, *18*, 1298–1309. [CrossRef] [PubMed]
44. Punde, T.H.; Wu, W.H.; Lien, P.C.; Chang, Y.L.; Kuo, P.H.; Chang, M.D.; Lee, K.Y.; Huang, C.D.; Kuo, H.P.; Chan, Y.F.; et al. A biologically inspired lung-on-a-chip device for the study of protein-induced lung inflammation. *Integr. Biol.* **2015**, *7*, 162–169. [CrossRef] [PubMed]
45. Nesmith, A.P.; Agarwal, A.; McCain, M.L.; Parker, K.K. Human airway musculature on a chip: An in vitro model of allergic asthmatic bronchoconstriction and bronchodilation. *Lab Chip* **2014**, *14*, 3925–3936. [CrossRef]
46. Huh, D.; Leslie, D.C.; Matthews, B.D.; Fraser, J.P.; Jurek, S.; Hamilton, G.A.; Thorneloe, K.S.; McAlexander, M.A.; Ingber, D.E. A human disease model of drug toxicity-induced pulmonary edema in a lung-on-a-chip microdevice. *Sci. Transl. Med.* **2012**, *4*, 159ra147. [CrossRef]
47. Zamprogno, P.; Wuthrich, S.; Achenbach, S.; Thoma, G.; Stucki, J.D.; Hobi, N.; Schneider-Daum, N.; Lehr, C.M.; Huwer, H.; Geiser, T.; et al. Second-generation lung-on-a-chip with an array of stretchable alveoli made with a biological membrane. *Commun. Biol.* **2021**, *4*, 1–10. [CrossRef]
48. Huang, D.; Liu, T.; Liao, J.; Maharjan, S.; Xie, X.; Perez, M.; Anaya, I.; Wang, S.; Tirado Mayer, A.; Kang, Z.; et al. Reversed-engineered human alveolar lung-on-a-chip model. *Proc. Natl. Acad. Sci. USA* **2021**, *118*. [CrossRef]
49. Zhang, M.; Xu, C.; Jiang, L.; Qin, J. A 3D human lung-on-a-chip model for nanotoxicity testing. *Toxicol. Res.* **2018**, *7*, 1048–1060. [CrossRef]
50. Xu, C.; Zhang, M.; Chen, W.; Jiang, L.; Chen, C.; Qin, J. Assessment of Air Pollutant PM2.5 Pulmonary Exposure Using a 3D Lung-on-Chip Model. *ACS Biomater. Sci. Eng.* **2020**, *6*, 3081–3090. [CrossRef]
51. Xu, Z.; Li, E.; Guo, Z.; Yu, R.; Hao, H.; Xu, Y.; Sun, Z.; Li, X.; Lyu, J.; Wang, Q. Design and Construction of a Multi-Organ Microfluidic Chip Mimicking the in vivo Microenvironment of Lung Cancer Metastasis. *ACS Appl. Mater. Interfaces* **2016**, *8*, 25840–25847. [CrossRef] [PubMed]
52. Srinivasan, B.; Kolli, A.R.; Esch, M.B.; Abaci, H.E.; Shuler, M.L.; Hickman, J.J. TEER measurement techniques for in vitro barrier model systems. *J. Lab. Autom.* **2015**, *20*, 107–126. [CrossRef]
53. Henry, O.Y.F.; Villenave, R.; Cronce, M.J.; Leineweber, W.D.; Benz, M.A.; Ingber, D.E. Organs-on-chips with integrated electrodes for trans-epithelial electrical resistance (TEER) measurements of human epithelial barrier function. *Lab Chip* **2017**, *17*, 2264–2271. [CrossRef]
54. Khalid, M.A.U.; Kim, Y.S.; Ali, M.; Lee, B.G.; Cho, Y.-J.; Choi, K.H. A lung cancer-on-chip platform with integrated biosensors for physiological monitoring and toxicity assessment. *Biochem. Eng. J.* **2020**, *155*, 107469. [CrossRef]
55. Mermoud, Y.; Felder, M.; Stucki, J.D.; Stucki, A.O.; Guenat, O.T. Microimpedance tomography system to monitor cell activity and membrane movements in a breathing lung-on-chip. *Sens. Actuators B Chem.* **2018**, *255*, 3647–3653. [CrossRef]
56. Stucki, A.O.; Stucki, J.D.; Hall, S.R.; Felder, M.; Mermoud, Y.; Schmid, R.A.; Geiser, T.; Guenat, O.T. A lung-on-a-chip array with an integrated bio-inspired respiration mechanism. *Lab Chip* **2015**, *15*, 1302–1310. [CrossRef]
57. Skardal, A.; Murphy, S.V.; Devarasetty, M.; Mead, I.; Kang, H.W.; Seol, Y.J.; Shrike Zhang, Y.; Shin, S.R.; Zhao, L.; Aleman, J.; et al. Multi-tissue interactions in an integrated three-tissue organ-on-a-chip platform. *Sci. Rep.* **2017**, *7*, 8837. [CrossRef]
58. Qiu, G.; Gai, Z.; Tao, Y.; Schmitt, J.; Kullak-Ublick, G.A.; Wang, J. Dual-Functional Plasmonic Photothermal Biosensors for Highly Accurate Severe Acute Respiratory Syndrome Coronavirus 2 Detection. *ACS Nano* **2020**, *14*, 5268–5277. [CrossRef] [PubMed]
59. Jin, C.E.; Lee, T.Y.; Koo, B.; Sung, H.; Kim, S.-H.; Shin, Y. Rapid virus diagnostic system using bio-optical sensor and microfluidic sample processing. *Sens. Actuators B Chem.* **2018**, *255*, 2399–2406. [CrossRef]
60. Fumet, J.-D.; Truntzer, C.; Yarchoan, M.; Ghiringhelli, F. Tumour mutational burden as a biomarker for immunotherapy: Current data and emerging concepts. *Eur. J. Cancer* **2020**, *131*, 40–50. [CrossRef]
61. Ballman, K.V. Biomarker: Predictive or Prognostic? *J. Clin. Oncol.* **2015**, *33*, 3968. [CrossRef]

62. Schwaederle, M.; Zhao, M.; Lee, J.J.; Lazar, V.; Leyland-Jones, B.; Schilsky, R.L.; Mendelsohn, J.; Kurzrock, R. Association of Biomarker-Based Treatment Strategies With Response Rates and Progression-Free Survival in Refractory Malignant Neoplasms AMeta-analysis. *JAMA Oncol.* **2016**, *2*, 1452–1459. [CrossRef]
63. Jayanthi, V.S.P.K.S.A.; Das, A.B.; Saxena, U. Recent advances in biosensor development for the detection of cancer biomarkers. *Biosens. Bioelectron.* **2017**, *91*, 15–23. [CrossRef]
64. Califf, R.M. Biomarker definitions and their applications. *Exp. Biol. Med.* **2018**, *243*, 213–221. [CrossRef] [PubMed]
65. Wu, L.; Qu, X. Cancer biomarker detection: Recent achievements and challenges. *Chem. Soc. Rev.* **2015**, *44*, 2963–2997. [CrossRef] [PubMed]
66. Bock, C.; Halbritter, F.; Carmona, F.J.; Tierling, S.; Datlinger, P.; Assenov, Y.; Berdasco, M.; Bergmann, A.K.; Booher, K.; Busato, F.; et al. Quantitative comparison of DNA methylation assays for biomarker development and clinical applications. *Nat. Biotechnol.* **2016**, *34*, 726. [CrossRef]
67. Koch, A.; Joosten, S.C.; Feng, Z.; de Ruijter, T.C.; Draht, M.X.; Melotte, V.; Smits, K.M.; Veeck, J.; Herman, J.G.; Van Neste, L.; et al. Analysis of DNA methylation in cancer: Location revisited. *Nat. Rev. Clin. Oncol.* **2018**, *15*, 459–466. [CrossRef] [PubMed]
68. Thind, A.; Wilson, C. Exosomal miRNAs as cancer biomarkers and therapeutic targets. *J. Extracell. Vesicles* **2016**, *5*. [CrossRef]
69. Condrat, C.E.; Thompson, D.C.; Barbu, M.G.; Bugnar, O.L.; Boboc, A.; Cretoiu, D.; Suciu, N.; Cretoiu, S.M.; Voinea, S.C. miRNAs as Biomarkers in Disease: Latest Findings Regarding Their Role in Diagnosis and Prognosis. *Cells* **2020**, *9*, 276. [CrossRef]
70. Ghrera, A.S.; Pandey, C.M.; Malhotra, B.D. Multiwalled carbon nanotube modified microfluidic-based biosensor chip for nucleic acid detection. *Sens. Actuators B Chem.* **2018**, *266*, 329–336. [CrossRef]
71. Roether, J.; Chu, K.-Y.; Willenbacher, N.; Shen, A.Q.; Bhalla, N. Real-time monitoring of DNA immobilization and detection of DNA polymerase activity by a microfluidic nanoplasmonic platform. *Biosens. Bioelectron.* **2019**, *142*. [CrossRef]
72. Dutta, G.; Rainbow, J.; Zupancic, U.; Papamatthaiou, S.; Estrela, P.; Moschou, D. Microfluidic Devices for Label-Free DNA Detection. *Chemosensors* **2018**, *6*, 43. [CrossRef]
73. Lu, T.X.; Rothenberg, M.E. MicroRNA. *J. Allergy Clin. Immunol.* **2018**, *141*, 1202–1207. [CrossRef] [PubMed]
74. Cohen, J.D.; Javed, A.A.; Thoburn, C.; Wong, F.; Tie, J.; Gibbs, P.; Schmidt, C.M.; Yip-Schneider, M.T.; Allen, P.J.; Schattner, M.; et al. Combined circulating tumor DNA and protein biomarker-based liquid biopsy for the earlier detection of pancreatic cancers. *Proc. Natl. Acad. Sci. USA* **2017**, *114*, 10202–10207. [CrossRef] [PubMed]
75. Arbour, K.C.; Riely, G.J. Systemic Therapy for Locally Advanced and Metastatic Non-Small Cell Lung Cancer A Review. *JAMA J. Am. Med. Assoc.* **2019**, *322*, 764–774. [CrossRef] [PubMed]
76. Prelaj, A.; Tay, R.; Ferrara, R.; Chaput, N.; Besse, B.; Califano, R. Predictive biomarkers of response for immune checkpoint inhibitors in non-small-cell lung cancer. *Eur. J. Cancer* **2019**, *106*, 144–159. [CrossRef] [PubMed]
77. Sheng, Y.; Zhang, T.H.; Zhang, S.H.; Johnston, M.; Zheng, X.H.; Shan, Y.Y.; Liu, T.; Huang, Z.N.; Qian, F.Y.; Xie, Z.H.; et al. A CRISPR/Cas13a-powered catalytic electrochemical biosensor for successive and highly sensitive RNA diagnostics. *Biosens. Bioelectron.* **2021**, *178*, 10. [CrossRef]
78. Portela, A.; Calvo-Lozano, O.; Estevez, M.C.; Escuela, A.M.; Lechuga, L.M. Optical nanogap antennas as plasmonic biosensors for the detection of miRNA biomarkers. *J. Mat. Chem. B* **2020**, *8*, 4310–4317. [CrossRef]
79. Aoki, H.; Torimura, M.; Nakazato, T. 384-Channel electrochemical sensor array chips based on hybridization-triggered switching for simultaneous oligonucleotide detection. *Biosens. Bioelectron.* **2019**, *136*, 76–83. [CrossRef]
80. Zeng, N.; Xiang, J. Detection of KRAS G12D point mutation level by anchor-like DNA electrochemical biosensor. *Talanta* **2019**, *198*, 111–117. [CrossRef]
81. Wu, Y.; Kwak, K.J.; Agarwal, K.; Marras, A.; Wang, C.; Mao, Y.; Huang, X.; Ma, J.; Yu, B.; Lee, R.; et al. Detection of Extracellular RNAs in Cancer and Viral Infection via Tethered Cationic Lipoplex Nanoparticles Containing Molecular Beacons. *Anal. Chem.* **2013**, *85*, 11265–11274. [CrossRef] [PubMed]
82. Chiu, N.F.; Yang, H.T. High-Sensitivity Detection of the Lung Cancer Biomarker CYFRA21-1 in Serum Samples Using a Carboxyl-MoS2 Functional Film for SPR-Based Immunosensors. *Front. Bioeng. Biotechnol.* **2020**, *8*, 14. [CrossRef] [PubMed]
83. Cheng, S.; Hideshima, S.; Kuroiwa, S.; Nakanishi, T.; Osaka, T. Label-free detection of tumor markers using field effect transistor (FET)-based biosensors for lung cancer diagnosis. *Sens. Actuators B Chem.* **2015**, *212*, 329–334. [CrossRef]
84. Zou, Y.; Zhang, X.; An, C.; Ran, C.; Ying, K.; Wang, P. A point-of-care testing system with Love-wave sensor and immunogold staining enhancement for early detection of lung cancer. *Biomed. Microdevices* **2014**, *16*, 927–935. [CrossRef] [PubMed]
85. Chakravarty, S.; Lai, W.-C.; Zou, Y.; Drabkin, H.A.; Gemmill, R.M.; Simon, G.R.; Chin, S.H.; Chen, R.T. Multiplexed specific label-free detection of NCI-H358 lung cancer cell line lysates with silicon based photonic crystal microcavity biosensors. *Biosens. Bioelectron.* **2013**, *43*, 50–55. [CrossRef]
86. Feng, J.; Wu, T.; Cheng, Q.; Ma, H.; Ren, X.; Wang, X.; Lee, J.Y.; Wei, Q.; Ju, H. A microfluidic cathodic photoelectrochemical biosensor chip for the targeted detection of cytokeratin 19 fragments 21-1. *Lab Chip* **2021**, *21*, 378–384. [CrossRef] [PubMed]
87. Washburn, A.L.; Shia, W.W.; Lenkeit, K.A.; Lee, S.-H.; Bailey, R.C. Multiplexed cancer biomarker detection using chip-integrated silicon photonic sensor arrays. *Analyst* **2016**, *141*, 5358–5365. [CrossRef]
88. Gao, Y.; Huo, W.; Zhang, L.; Lian, J.; Tao, W.; Song, C.; Tang, J.; Shi, S.; Gao, Y. Multiplex measurement of twelve tumor markers using a GMR multi-biomarker immunoassay biosensor. *Biosens. Bioelectron.* **2019**, *123*, 204–210. [CrossRef]
89. Gao, A.; Yang, X.; Tong, J.; Zhou, L.; Wang, Y.; Zhao, J.; Mao, H.; Li, T. Multiplexed detection of lung cancer biomarkers in patients serum with CMOS-compatible silicon nanowire arrays. *Biosens. Bioelectron.* **2017**, *91*, 482–488. [CrossRef]

90. Zhang, Y.; Liu, Y.; Liu, H.; Tang, W.H. Exosomes: Biogenesis, biologic function and clinical potential. *Cell Biosci.* **2019**, *9*. [CrossRef] [PubMed]
91. Tai, Y.-L.; Chen, K.-C.; Hsieh, J.-T.; Shen, T.-L. Exosomes in cancer development and clinical applications. *Cancer Sci.* **2018**, *109*, 2364–2374. [CrossRef]
92. Yu, W.; Hurley, J.; Roberts, D.; Chakrabortty, S.K.; Enderle, D.; Noerholm, M.; Breakefield, X.O.; Skog, J.K. Exosome-based liquid biopsies in cancer: Opportunities and challenges. *Ann. Oncol.* **2021**, *32*, 466–477. [CrossRef]
93. Yang, Q.; Cheng, L.; Hu, L.; Lou, D.; Zhang, T.; Li, J.; Zhu, Q.; Liu, F. An integrative microfluidic device for isolation and ultrasensitive detection of lung cancer-specific exosomes from patient urine. *Biosens. Bioelectron.* **2020**, *163*, 112290. [CrossRef]
94. Chen, H.; Zhang, Z.; Liu, H.; Zhang, Z.; Lin, C.; Wang, B. Hybrid magnetic and deformability based isolation of circulating tumor cells using microfluidics. *AIP Adv.* **2019**, *9*, 025023. [CrossRef]
95. Nguyen, N.V.; Jen, C.P. Impedance detection integrated with dielectrophoresis enrichment platform for lung circulating tumor cells in a microfluidic channel. *Biosens. Bioelectron.* **2018**, *121*, 10–18. [CrossRef]
96. Ngoc-Viet, N.; Yang, C.-H.; Liu, C.-I.; Kuo, C.-H.; Wu, D.-C.; Jen, C.-P. An Aptamer-Based Capacitive Sensing Platform for Specific Detection of Lung Carcinoma Cells in the Microfluidic Chip. *Biosensors* **2018**, *8*, 98. [CrossRef]
97. Nabovati, G.; Ghafar-Zadeh, E.; Letourneau, A.; Sawan, M. Towards High Throughput Cell Growth Screening: A New CMOS 8 × 8 Biosensor Array for Life Science Applications. *IEEE Trans. Biomed. Circuits Syst.* **2017**, *11*, 380–391. [CrossRef] [PubMed]
98. Do, L.Q.; Thuy, H.T.T.; Bui, T.T.; Dau, V.T.; Nguyen, N.V.; Duc, T.C.; Jen, C.P. Dielectrophoresis Microfluidic Enrichment Platform with Built-In Capacitive Sensor for Rare Tumor Cell Detection. *BioChip J.* **2018**, *12*, 114–122. [CrossRef]
99. Li, Y.; Xu, T.; Zou, H.; Chen, X.; Sun, D.; Yang, M. Cell migration microfluidics for electrotaxis-based heterogeneity study of lung cancer cells. *Biosens. Bioelectron.* **2017**, *89*, 837–845. [CrossRef] [PubMed]
100. Pan, Y.; Jiang, D.; Gu, C.; Qiu, Y.; Wan, H.; Wang, P. 3D microgroove electrical impedance sensing to examine 3D cell cultures for antineoplastic drug assessment. *Microsyst. Nanoeng.* **2020**, *6*, 1–10. [CrossRef]
101. Noh, S.; Kim, H. In-air EIS sensor for in situ and real-time monitoring of in vitro epithelial cells under air-exposure. *Lab Chip* **2020**, *20*, 1751–1761. [CrossRef]
102. Zirath, H.; Rothbauer, M.; Spitz, S.; Bachmann, B.; Jordan, C.; Muller, B.; Ehgartner, J.; Priglinger, E.; Muhleder, S.; Redl, H.; et al. Every Breath You Take: Non-invasive Real-Time Oxygen Biosensing in Two- and Three-Dimensional Microfluidic Cell Models. *Front. Physiol.* **2018**, *9*, 815. [CrossRef]
103. Zhao, X.; Gao, W.; Yin, J.; Fan, W.; Wang, Z.; Hu, K.; Mai, Y.; Luan, A.; Xu, B.; Jin, Q. A high-precision thermometry microfluidic chip for real-time monitoring of the physiological process of live tumour cells. *Talanta* **2021**, *226*, 122101. [CrossRef]
104. Lafleur, J.P.; Joensson, A.; Senkbeil, S.; Kutter, J.P. Recent advances in lab-on-a-chip for biosensing applications. *Biosens. Bioelectron.* **2016**, *76*, 213–233. [CrossRef]
105. Luka, G.; Ahmadi, A.; Najjaran, H.; Alocilja, E.; DeRosa, M.; Wolthers, K.; Malki, A.; Aziz, H.; Althani, A.; Hoorfar, M. Microfluidics Integrated Biosensors: A Leading Technology towards Lab-on-a-Chip and Sensing Applications. *Sensors* **2015**, *15*, 30011–30031. [CrossRef]
106. Kumar, S.; Kumar, S.; Ali, M.A.; Anand, P.; Agrawal, V.V.; John, R.; Maji, S.; Malhotra, B.D. Microfluidic-integrated biosensors: Prospects for point-of-care diagnostics. *Biotechnol. J.* **2013**, *8*, 1267–1279. [CrossRef] [PubMed]
107. Loo, J.F.C.; Ho, A.H.P.; Turner, A.P.F.; Mak, W.C. Integrated Printed Microfluidic Biosensors. *Trends Biotechnol.* **2019**, *37*, 1104–1120. [CrossRef]
108. Khan, N.I.; Song, E. Lab-on-a-Chip Systems for Aptamer-Based Biosensing. *Micromachines* **2020**, *11*. [CrossRef]
109. Liu, Y.; Zhang, X. Microfluidics-Based Plasmonic Biosensing System Based on Patterned Plasmonic Nanostructure Arrays. *Micromachines* **2021**, *12*, 826. [CrossRef] [PubMed]
110. Liu, D.; Wang, J.; Wu, L.; Huang, Y.; Zhang, Y.; Zhu, M.; Wang, Y.; Zhu, Z.; Yang, C. Trends in miniaturized biosensors for point-of-care testing. *TrAC—Trends Anal. Chem.* **2020**, *122*. [CrossRef]
111. Derkus, B. Applying the miniaturization technologies for biosensor design. *Biosens. Bioelectron.* **2016**, *79*, 901–913. [CrossRef] [PubMed]

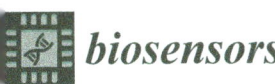

Review

Biodegradable Metal Organic Frameworks for Multimodal Imaging and Targeting Theranostics

Xiangdong Lai, Hui Jiang and Xuemei Wang *

State Key Laboratory of Bioelectronics (Chien-Shiung Wu Lab), School of Biological Science and Medical Engineering, Southeast University, Nanjing 210096, China; ab58472416@163.com (X.L.); sungi@seu.edu.cn (H.J.)
* Correspondence: xuewang@seu.edu.cn; Tel.: +86-25-83792177

Abstract: Though there already had been notable progress in developing efficient therapeutic strategies for cancers, there still exist many requirements for significant improvement of the safety and efficiency of targeting cancer treatment. Thus, the rational design of a fully biodegradable and synergistic bioimaging and therapy system is of great significance. Metal organic framework (MOF) is an emerging class of coordination materials formed from metal ion/ion clusters nodes and organic ligand linkers. It arouses increasing interest in various areas in recent years. The unique features of adjustable composition, porous and directional structure, high specific surface areas, biocompatibility, and biodegradability make it possible for MOFs to be utilized as nano-drugs or/and nanocarriers for multimodal imaging and therapy. This review outlines recent advances in developing MOFs for multimodal treatment of cancer and discusses the prospects and challenges ahead.

Keywords: biodegradable materials; metal-organic framework; metal ion nodes; multimode imaging; theranostic nano-platforms

1. Introduction

Cancer has been a serious threat to human health [1]. The accurate therapy of cancer still needs to overcome many great difficulties [2,3]. Each therapy, such as chemotherapy (CT), chemo-dynamic therapy (CDT), radiation therapy (RT), radio-dynamic therapy (RDT), microwave thermal therapy (MTT), microwave dynamic therapy (MDT), photothermal therapy (PTT), and photodynamic therapy (PDT), has its inherent advantages and defects [4–6]. Hence, the treatment of cancers has gradually developed from the past monotherapy mode to the current multimode synergistic therapy to enhance therapeutic effects. With the rapid development of nanotechnology, the realization of multimode synergistic therapy depends largely on how to integrate multiple treatment modes into a single nano-platform rather than purely carrying out physical mixing to obtain a simple additive treatment effect. In recent years, emerging and rapidly developing MOF materials have shown enormous potential in multimodal synergistic therapy because of their unique porous structure and characteristics. MOF is a kind of organic inorganic hybrid material through coordination bonds formation between metal ion/ion clusters nodes and organic ligand linkers [7–11]. MOF characterizes by variable compositions and structures, adjustable porosity and pore sizes, high surface areas, good biocompatibility, and biodegradability [7,12,13]. Weak coordination bonds can endow MOFs with a stable but degradable structure [14–16]. Nanoscale pores and an ordered crystal structure allow MOFs to accumulate in tumor through enhanced permeability and retention effect (EPR) [17,18]. At the same time, the organic linker can be additionally functionalized for targeting cancer therapy [19,20]. Furthermore, the good dispersibility and biocompatibility of specific MOFs can ensure the biosafety of targeting treatment in vivo [21]. Adjustable composition results in controlled synthesis with different morphology, size, and chemical properties, making MOF itself a nano-drug for multimodal imaging and therapy by choosing appropriate metal nodes and organic ligands [22,23]. Moreover, the porous and ordered

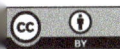

structure and the high ratio surface areas are suitable for efficient loading of various cargos for multimodal imaging and therapy [24–28]. MOF-based nanomaterials were applied to fluorescence imaging (FL) [29–32], photoacoustic imaging (PAI) [33], magnetic resonance imaging (MRI) [34–36], computed tomography imaging (CTI) [37–39], photothermal imaging (PTI) [40,41] and positron emission tomography (PET) imaging [42–45]. It is worth mentioning that multimodal imaging [46–52] is beneficial for tumor diagnosis and accurate position. MOF-based heterogeneous hybridization may serve as an effective methodology for multimodal imaging and synergistic therapy. It integrates the advantages of various materials and endues the hybrid materials with whole new physicochemical properties, realizing theranostic nano-platforms through multimode imaging-guided therapy. In this review, the development of biodegradable MOFs as nano-drugs and nanocarriers for multimodal imaging and therapy in recent years will be summarized and discussed, as shown in Figure 1, and the prospects and challenges of MOFs in multimodal synergistic treatment will also be explored for promising clinic/biomedical applications.

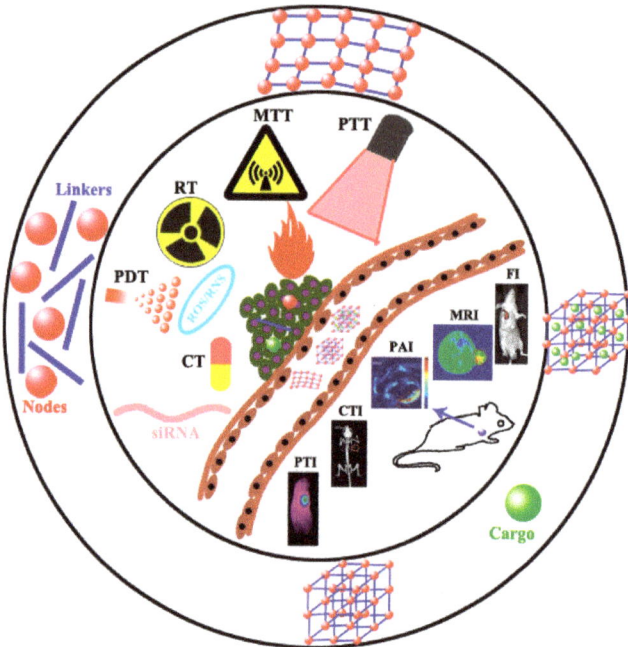

Figure 1. Schematic diagram of MOFs as nano-drugs and nanocarriers for multimodal theranostic, typically comprising a suitable and effective combination of CT, CDT, RT, RDT, PTT, PDT, MDT, MTT, gas therapy and gene therapy, and imaging of FI, MRI, PAI, CTI and PTI.

2. MOFs as Nano-Drugs

Due to the nearly infinite combination of metal ion/ion clusters nodes and organic ligand linkers, the physical and chemical properties of MOFs could be regulated for many applications. Through careful selection and design, metal ion/ion clusters nodes and organic ligand linkers can be directly and fully utilized as nano-drugs to realize multimodal imaging and therapy. Liu et al. [53] reported a nanoscale MOF synthesized by hafnium (Hf^{4+}) and tetra (4-carboxyphenyl) porphyrin (TCPP), in which TCPP as a photosensitizer converted tissue oxygen to cytotoxic singlet oxygen under light irradiation and could be used for PDT. At the same time, Hf^{4+} characterized by strong X-ray absorption capacity could act as a radiation sensitizer to enhance RT. Compared to other metals with a higher atomic number, Hf was relatively safe and showed no apparent biological toxicity. Hf-TCPP MOF was biodegradable and easily removed from the mouse body. Hf-TCPP MOF as a biodegradable carrier-free system was used for combined RT and PDT in vitro and in vivo, demonstrating a remarkable anti-tumor effect. Lin's group [54] reported Cu-TBP (5,10,15,20-tetrabenzoatoporphyrin) nanoscale MOF mediated synergistic hormone-induced CDT and light-induced PDT in the tumor model with high estradiol expression. The degradable Cu-TBP MOFs were accumulated in tumor cells efficiently and decomposed into Cu^{2+} and H_4TBP by monitoring free porphyrin fluorescence, which was entirely quenched by the paramagnetic Cu^{2+} in intact MOF at pH 7.4 and reappeared in acid tumor cell microenvironment due to the decomposition of Cu-TBP (Figure 2A). Cu-TBP was injected into dorsal subcutaneous tumors and produced Cu^{2+} and porphyrin in the low pH tumor microenvironment. Cu^{2+} ions, as redox-active metal centers, catalyzed estradiol metabolism to generate hydrogen peroxide, hydroxyl radical (·OH), superoxide (O^{2-}) species, and other ROS for CDT, whereas H_4TBP mediated light-induced PDT. This MOF-mediated radical treatment depleted intratumoral estradiol and inhibited tumor growth. Upon light irradiation, H_4TBP produced ROS to destroy the irradiated cancer cells, causing immunogenic cell death and tumor antigens release. Released tumor antigens and injected PD-L1 antibody caused the effective T cell proliferation and infiltration into the tumor, overcoming the immunosuppressive tumor microenvironment and simultaneously effectively inhibiting the growth of distant tumors (Figure 2B).

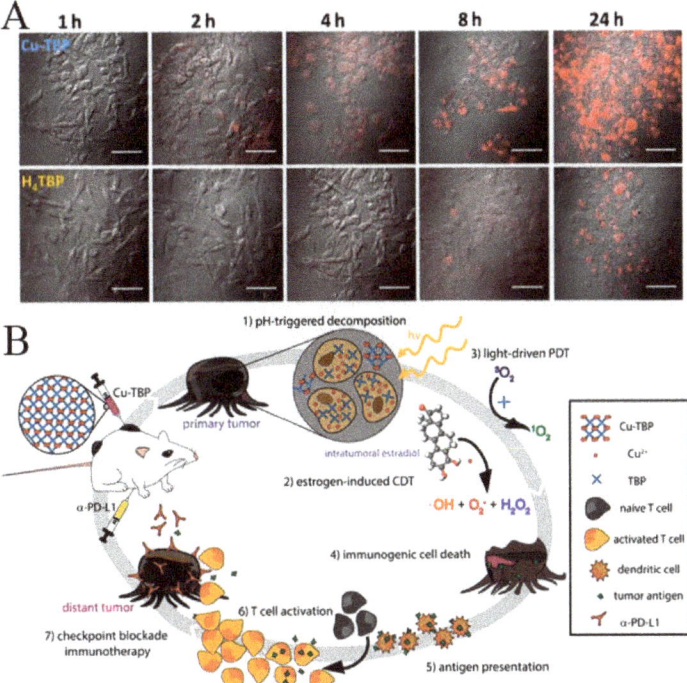

Figure 2. (**A**) B16F10 cellular uptake of Cu-TBP or H_4TBP at different time-points after incubation with equivalent TBP concentrations of 20 mM observed by confocal imaging. Free H_4TBP emits red fluorescence. Scale bar, 50 µm. (**B**) Synergy of Cu-TBP mediated radical therapy stimulated by hormone, light and checkpoint blockade immunotherapy. Reprinted with permission from Ref. [54]. Copyright 2019, Elsevier.

Zirconium(IV) chloride ($ZrCl_4$), Manganese(II) chloride tetrahydrate, and 1,4-Benzenedicarboxylic acid (H_2BDC) were used as raw materials to chemically synthesize Mn-doped

Zr MOF by a one-pot hydrothermal method [55]. The flexible and microporous structure is beneficial to the strongly confined inelastic collision of ions, resulting in a significant microwave thermal conversion efficiency as high as 28.7%. The Mn-ZrMOF catalyzed the degradation of H_2O_2 to generate ·OH under MW irradiation. The in vitro and in vivo experimental studies confirmed that a union of MTT and MDT with simultaneous generation of heat and ROS under mild MW irradiation realized synergistic inhibition of the growth of tumors, as schematically reported in Figure 3. The Mn-ZrMOF was degradable in vivo and excreted out of the body gradually, demonstrating that it is a bio-safe therapeutic nano-agent.

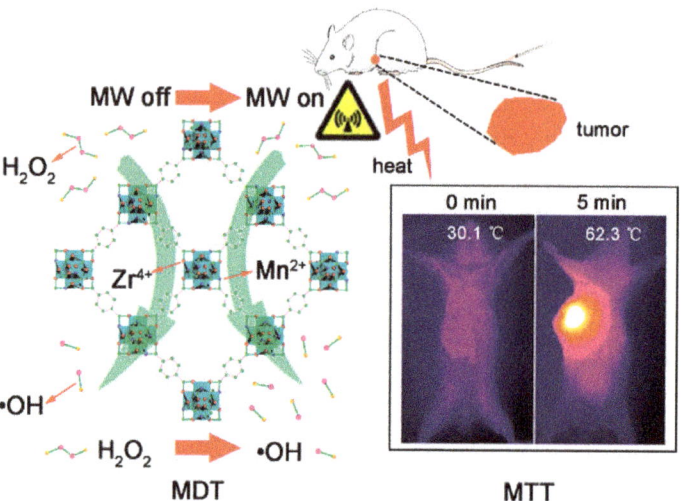

Figure 3. Mn-Zr MOF generates abundant ROS of ·OH and a high microwave thermal conversion efficiency after exposure to MW irradiation, resulting in efficiently inhibiting the cancerous cell growth through the synergic effect of MDT and MTT. Reprinted with permission from Ref. [55]. Copyright 2018, American Chemical Society.

Lan et al. [56] reported two MOF nanolayers, Hf_{12}-Ir, and Hf_6-Ir (namely Iridium), schematically reported in Figure 4. Under X-ray irradiation, electron-dense Hf_{12} and Hf_6 secondary building units not only generated ·OH to enhance RT but also transferred energy to photosensitizing Ir (2,2'-bipyridine) [2-(2,4-difluorophenyl)-5-(trifluoromethyl) pyridine]$_2^+$ to generate single oxygen ($^1O_2$) and O_2^-, resulting in RDT. RT and RDT exerted superb anticancer effects at shallow X-ray doses.

Wu et al. prepared Cu-TCPP MOF nanosheets for dual-modal PTT and PDT. Upon 808 nm laser irradiation, the coexisting Cu^+ and Cu^{2+} exhibited excellent photothermal performance due to the strong near-infrared (NIR) absorption [41]. In the meantime, TCPP produced $^1O_2$ for PDT. The toxicity experiment indicated that Cu-TCPP has good biocompatibility. Due to Cu(II) in the Cu-TCPP nanosheets, near-infrared thermal imaging and T1-weighted magnetic resonance imaging (MRI) could be used to realize simultaneous diagnosis and therapy (Figure 5).

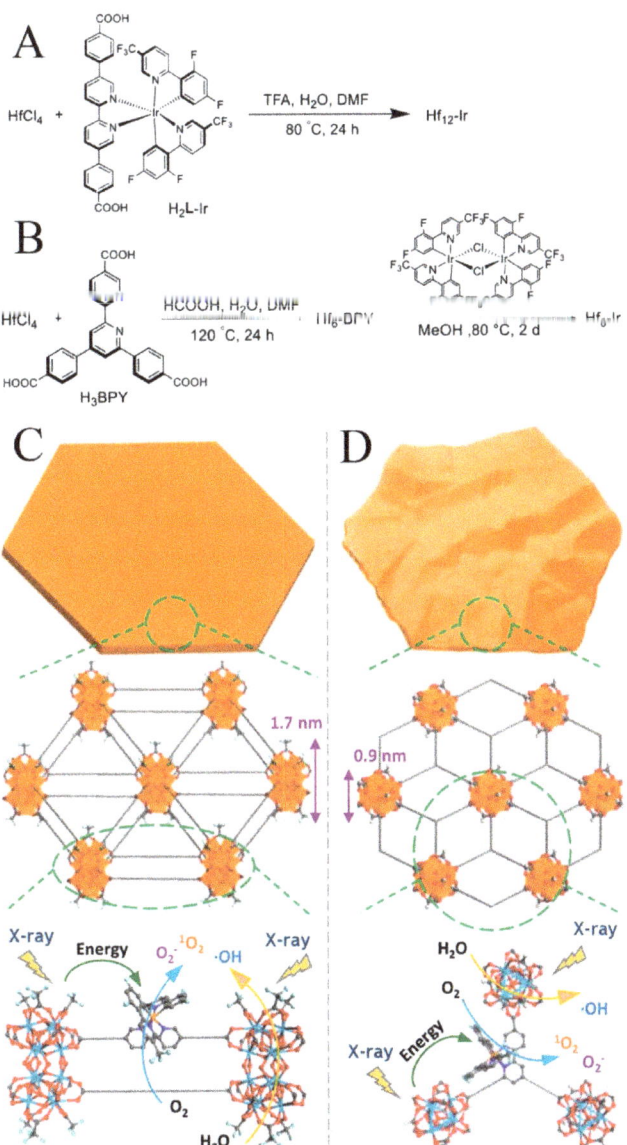

Figure 4. The synthesis methods, morphologies and structures of Hf$_{12}$-Ir MOF nanolayer (**A,C**) and Hf$_6$-Ir MOF nanolayer (**B,D**) and X-ray induced ROS generation. Reprinted with permission from Ref. [56]. Copyright 2018, American Chemical Society.

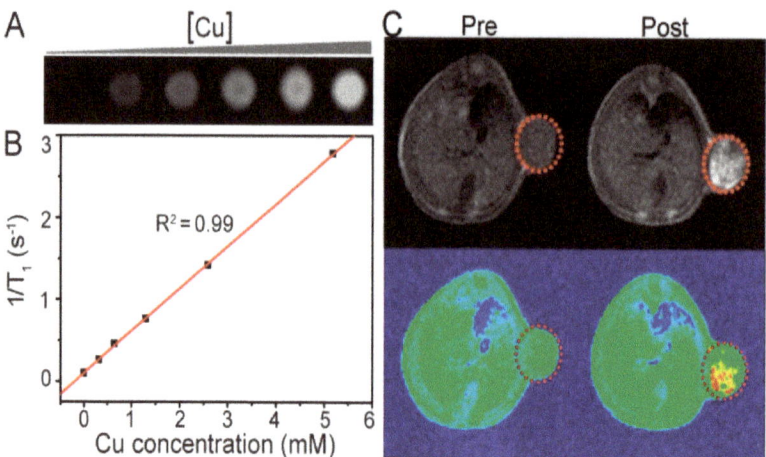

Figure 5. (**A**) MRI of the Cu-TCPP aqueous solution with different concentrations. (**B**) Plots of the 1/T1 value of the Cu-TCPP under concentration dependence. (**C**) mouse MRI before and after intratumoral injection of the Cu-TCPP. Red circles indicate the position of the tumor. Reprinted with permission from Ref. [41]. Copyright 2018, Ivyspring International Publisher.

3. MOFs as Nanocarriers

The porous and ordered structure, tunable sizes, and the high ratio surface areas make MOF easy to be loaded a variety of cargos efficiently and increase the cargo capacity. In 2006, Patricia first reported a MOF for drug delivery named Materials of Institute Lavoisier 100 and 101 (MIL-100 and 101) [57]. After more than ten years of rapid development, MOF was used to carry oxygen [58], chemotherapeutic agents [59], photosensitizer [60], photothermal conversion agents [15,61], Nucleic acids and proteins [62–65]. Du et al. [66] reported an intelligent stimuli-responsive and completely degradable MOF delivery system. Based on a "framework exchange" strategy, black phosphorous quantum dots (BPQDs) were embedded into ZIF-8 nanoparticles, which were used as sacrificial templates to prepare BP@HKUST-1 (BH). MIL-100(Fe) shell enveloped the BH core to form the core-shell structure, while s-nitroso-glutathione was encapsulated into HKUST-1@MIL-100. In tumor cells, the high levels of glutathione and ROS triggered the decomposition of s-nitroso-glutathione to produce NO and ·OH, causing the damage of mitochondria and DNA in tumor cells. Black phosphorus has superb biocompatibility and very high photothermal conversion efficiency. This MOF was fluorescent and photoacoustically active (Figure 6), allowing it to readily achieve accurate multiple therapies that use gas, free radicals, and PTT. Notably, this nanosystem completely degraded into phosphate radicals, terephthalic acid, and metal ions excreted out of the body.

He et al. fabricated a MOF consisting of Zr^{6+} nodes and TCPP ligand [67]. The gold nanoparticles (AuNPs) were decorated on the surface of MOF, which was conducive to effectively stabilize the nanostructure and increased radiotherapy sensitivity. Meanwhile, chemotherapeutic drug doxorubicin (Dox) was encapsulated into the MOF. The fabricated MOFs were densely packed polyethylene glycol (PEG) corona to form Dox@MOF-Au-PEG. Dox@MOF-Au-PEG oxygenated tumor microenvironment by catalyzing the degradation of H_2O_2 in tumor into O_2, resulting in enhancing O_2-dependent radiotherapy. Dox@MOF-Au-PEG combined the radiotherapy sensitization effect of AuNPs and the anticancer effect of Dox, achieving synergistic chemoradiotherapy, as shown in Figure 7. The stronger coordination interaction between phosphate ion and zirconium made the MOF readily decompose in PBS (2 mM), resulting in the burst release of porphyrin ligands and structural collapse. Once MOF was internalized by cancer cells, the phosphate in high concentration led to the disassembly of the NPs.

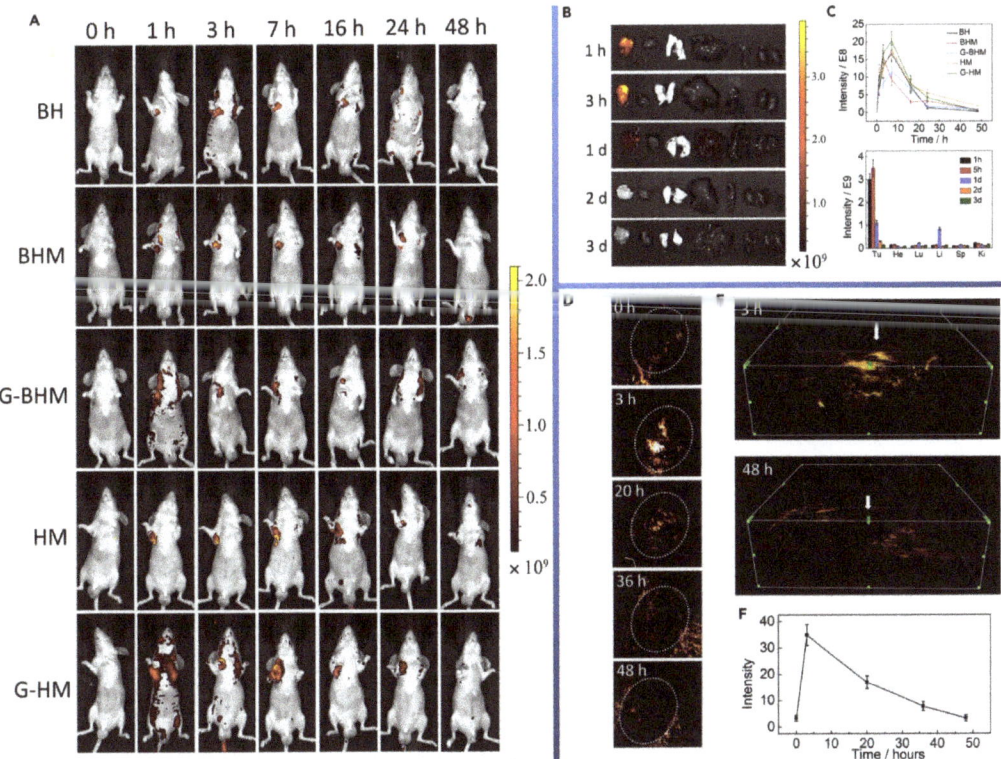

Figure 6. (**A**) Fluorescence imaging of SGC-7901 tumor-bearing model mice after intravenous injection of different materials at 7 time points. Unit of scale bar: $(p/s/cm^2/sr)/(mW/cm^2)$. (**B**) Ex vivo Fluorescence imaging of tumor, heart, lung, liver, spleen, and kidney in sequence in SGC-7901 tumor-bearing model mice after intravenous injection of G-BHM at 5 different time points. (**C**) Time-dependent in vivo integrated FL intensity for different materials (top) and in different organs (bottom). (**D**) PA imaging of SGC-7901 tumor after injection of G-BHM at different time points. (**E**) Stereoscopic PA images, and white arrow represents tumor zone. (**F**) PA signal intensity variation corresponding to part (**D**). Reprinted with permission from Ref. [66]. Copyright 2019, Elsevier Inc.

Zhang et al. [46] prepared a porous zirconium-ferriporphyrin MOF nano-shuttles (Zr-FeP) made from $ZrOCl_2 \cdot 8H_2O$ and $H_4TBP\text{-}Fe$, carrying the siRNA of 70 kDa heat shock protein (HSP70). Under NIR lasers, the siRNA/Zr-FeP MOF catalyzed endogenous H_2O_2 and O_2 to become $\cdot OH$ and $^1O_2$, while it had high photothermal conversion efficiency up to around 34%. Moreover, siRNA reversed the HSP70-mediated thermotherapy resistance, achieving PTT at a lower-temperature and avoiding the nearby normal tissues from the nonspecific thermal radiation damage. The siRNA/Zr-FeP significantly suppressed the tumor cell growth in vitro and in vivo through the synergistic effect of PTT at a lower temperature and PDT, shown in Figure 8. siRNA/Zr-FeP was effectively cleared out of the organism, via its gradual decomposition into small molecules and ions. Meanwhile, MOF nano-shuttles achieved PAI, CTI, and photothermal imaging (PTI) tri-mode tumor-specific imaging capability, providing a powerful theranostic tool for tumors.

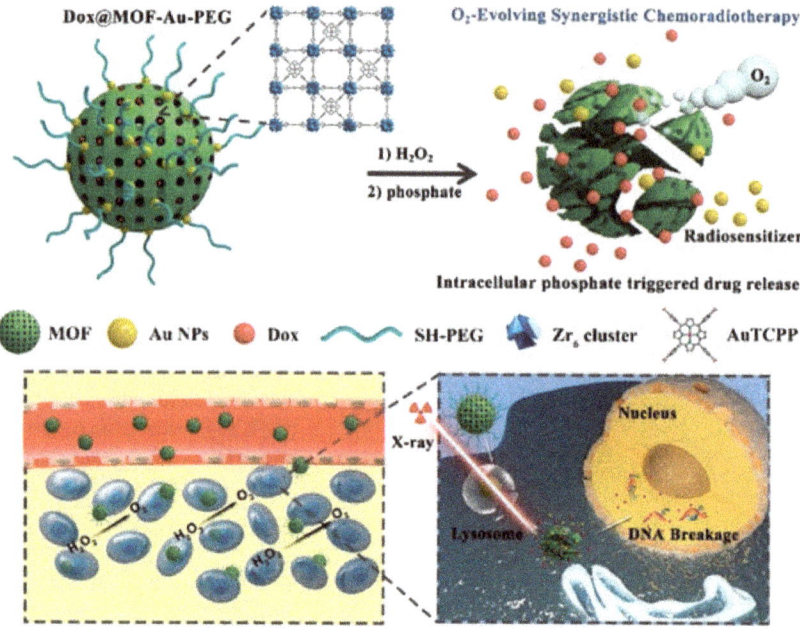

Figure 7. The structure of Dox@MOF-Au-PEG and the underlying of O_2-generating synergistic chemoradiotherapy Reprinted with permission from Ref. [67]. Copyright 2019, Wiley-VCH Verlag GmbH & Co. KGaA, Weinheim.

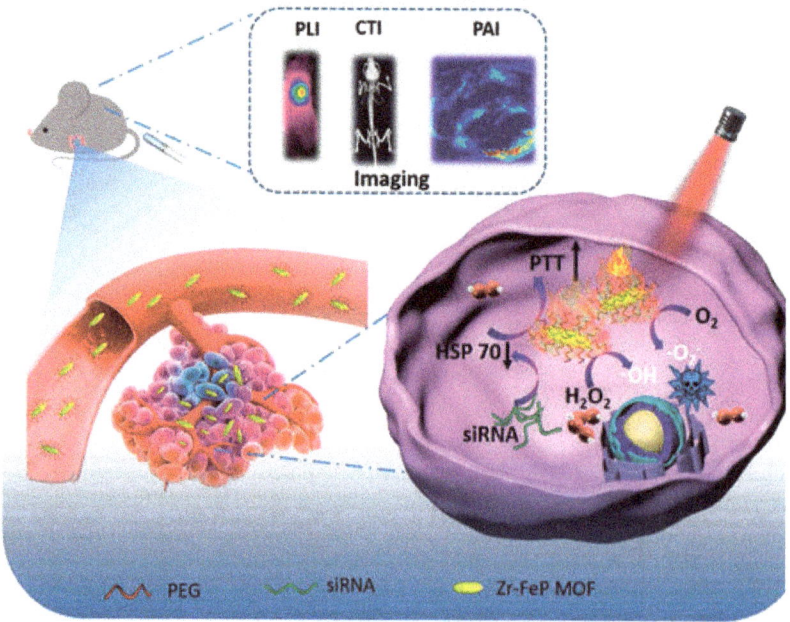

Figure 8. siRNA/Zr-FeP MOF mediates PTT at a lower temperature and PDT for cancer. Reprinted with permission from Ref. [46]. Copyright 2018, Elsevier B.V.

Liu et al. [68] encapsulated BPQDs and catalase into MIL-101 inner and outer layers, respectively, and constructed a MOF heterostructure, BPQDs-MIL@catalase-MIL. BPQDs exhibited two abilities of photothermal conversion for PTT and $^1O_2$ production for PDT. The catalase in the outer layer catalyzed H_2O_2 into O_2. O_2 was then converted into $^1O_2$ by BPQDs in the inner layer. The PDT/PTT synergistic therapy accelerated cancer cell apoptosis. Ni et al. [69] reported a Hf-DBB-Ru MOF consisting of Hf^{4+} and bis(2,2'-bipyridine) [5,5'-di(4-benzoate)-2,2'-bipyridine] ruthenium chloride for mitochondrial-targeted RDT and RT. Ru endowed Hf-DBB-Ru with strong mitochondria-targeted ability. Hf clusters generated abundant ·OH, and Ru-based linkers produced $^1O_2$ at low dose X-ray irradiation with high penetration. Yang et al. [70] developed cypate@MIL-53 nanoparticles. Fe^{3+} metal ions and the carboxyl group of cypate interacted to form precursor complexes, improving bioavailability and protecting the cypate NIR dye from photobleaching. Organic linkers H_2BDC coordinated with Fe^{3+} to generate crystallized MOFs. PEG and transferrin were functionalized on the surface of cypate@MIL-53 to enhance biocompatibility and tumor targeted functions. Cypate molecules gave this MOF the ability to behave as photosensitizers and photothermal agents for PDT and PTT, as shown in Figure 9. This MOF realized tumor targeted multimodal imaging (Near-infrared fluorescence images, PAI, and MRI).

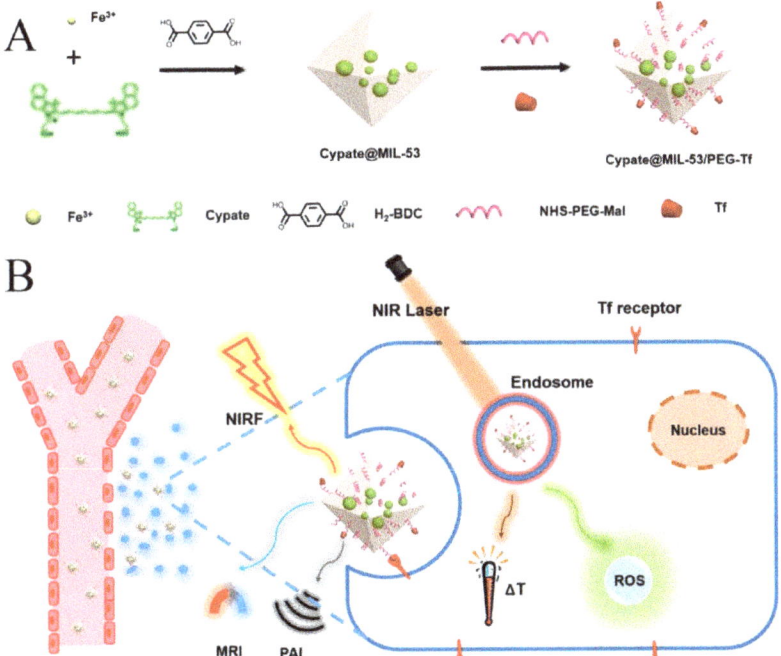

Figure 9. (A) the preparation of Cypate@MIL-53/PEG-Transferrin MOF composite and (B) its bioapplication for PDT and PTT. Reprinted with permission from Ref. [70]. Copyright 2019, American Chemical Society.

Chen et al. synthesized MIL-100 (Fe) coated Mn-based Prussian blue (PB) analogue (K_2Mn[Fe(CN)$_6$]), named as PBAM, by simply stirring and heating, losing photothermal activity of PB and T1-weighted MRI due to local confinement of Mn^{2+} [20]. In the mildly acidic tumor microenvironment, the MIL-100 shell was degraded, and the released Fe^{3+} exchanged with Mn^{2+} to synthesize in situ the more stable PB, Fe^{3+}–[Fe(CN)6]$^{4-}$, and to release free Mn^{2+}. Mn^{2+} reacted with endogenous H_2O_2 and HCO_3^- and generated ·OH for CDT. The excellent PAI and PTT of PB, and T1-weighted MRI and CDT of Mn^{2+} showed accurate theranostic effects (Figure 10).

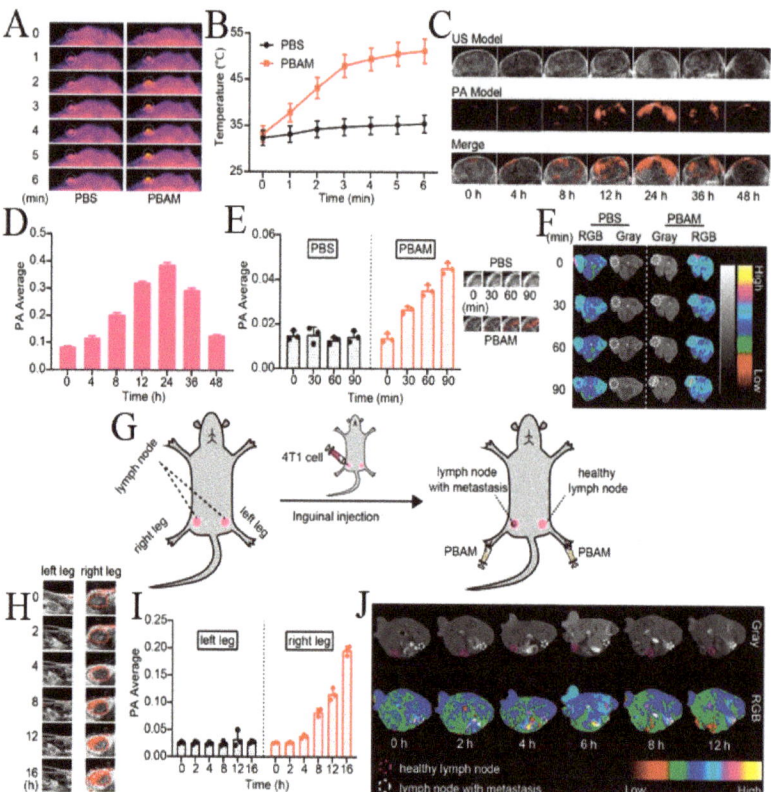

Figure 10. (A) Infrared thermal imaging and (B) tumor temperature of 4T1-tumor model mice after intravenous injection with PBAM under 808 nm laser (1 W cm^{-2}). White circle: tumor tissue. (C) Tumor PAI and (D) Corresponding PAI signal intensity of 4T1-tumor model mice after intravenous injection with PBAM. (E) Tumor PA signal intensity and corresponding PAI of 4T1-tumor model mice after subcutaneous injection with PBAM. (F) MRI of 4T1-tumor model mice after subcutaneous injection with PBAM. White circle: tumor tissue. (G) Schematic of lymphatic metastasis tumor model. (H) PAI of lymph nodes with or without metastasis at different time points after injection with PBAM. White circle: the lymph nodes in left leg. Red circle: the lymph nodes in right leg. (I) Corresponding PAI signal intensity of lymph nodes with or without metastasis. (J) MRI of lymph nodes with or without metastasis at different time points after injection with PBAM. Reprinted with permission from Ref. [20]. Copyright 2020, WILEY-VCH Verlag GmbH & Co. KGaA, Weinheim.

4. Summary and Perspectives

Weak coordination bonds result in degradable structures, which is very good for biomedical applications of MOFs. Furthermore, it is of great significance to develop MOFs as nano-drugs for multimodal imaging and therapy. MOFs itself as nano-drugs characterize by simplicity and efficiency, high drug loading, and lower dosages of node and linker drugs, benefiting for achieving expected anti-tumor effects and reducing toxic effects on normal tissues and cells. MOF specific features, such as flexible and diversified morphologies, tunable sizes, high surface areas, and tunable pore diameter make MOFs intelligent nanocarriers for multimodal diagnosis and therapy, easy to be loaded with a variety of cargos efficiently and harbor increased cargo capacity. To sum up, we have reviewed in detail the recent progress of biodegradable MOFs for multimodal theranostic, typically comprising a suitable and effective combination of CT, CDT, RT, RDT, PTT, PDT, MDT, MTT, gas therapy, and gene therapy, and imaging of FI, MRI, PAI, CTI, and PTI.

The efficacy of single modal therapy is often not ideal due to multidrug resistance, nonspecific heating, hypoxia, and other serious adverse effects. Though MOFs for multimodal therapy have demonstrated synergistic and enhanced therapeutic efficacy and low cytotoxicity in laboratory research, there is still great room for improvements to realize targeted cancer therapy. Firstly, most excellent researches lacked long-term experiments on the toxicity of MOFs. Comprehensive studies on the absorption, biodistribution, metabolism, excretion, clearance, and long-term tissue accumulation of MOFs are necessary for determining toxicity in vivo. Toxicity is effectively prevented through choosing highly biocompatible metal ions as nodes (e.g., Ca, Fe, Zn, etc.) and endogenous bioactive molecules as ligands [71,72]. The additional loaded cargo needs to be considered as well because of probable threats to the organism. In addition, there is an ever growing need for extensive and in-depth research on the mechanisms and pathways of MOFs degradation in vivo. This is due to the fact that current single imaging methods are not sufficient to monitor and recognize the degradation process of MOFs. Finally, current studies mainly focused on dual-modal therapy [73–77], while very few reports on tri- or more modal therapies were based on MOFs, demonstrating a more effective therapy. In brief, despite facing these challenges, a significant effort has been made to develop biodegradable MOFs for multimodal imaging and therapy, which can realize clinical translations and other bio-applications in the future.

Author Contributions: Conceptualization, X.L., H.J. and X.W.; writing—original draft preparation, X.L., H.J. and X.W.; writing—review and editing, X.L., H.J. and X.W.; visualization, X.L., H.J. and X.W.; supervision, X.W.; funding acquisition, X.W. All authors have read and agreed to the published version of the manuscript.

Funding: This work was supported by the National Natural Science Foundation of China (82061148012, 82027806, 91753106), the National Key Research and Development Program of China (2017YFA0205300), and Primary Research & Development Plan of Jiangsu Province (BE2019716).

Institutional Review Board Statement: Not applicable.

Informed Consent Statement: Not applicable.

Data Availability Statement: Not applicable.

Conflicts of Interest: The authors declare no conflict of interest.

References

1. Allmani, C.; Matsuda, T.; Di Carlo, V.; Harewood, R.; Matz, M.; Niksic, M.; Bonaventure, A.; Valkov, M.; Johnson, C.J.; Esteve, J.; et al. Global surveillance of trends in cancer survival 2000–14 (CONCORD-3): Analysis of individual records for 37 513 025 patients diagnosed with one of 18 cancers from 322 population-based registries in 71 countries. *Lancet* **2018**, *391*, 1023–1075. [CrossRef]
2. Li, S.; Jiang, Q.; Liu, S.; Zhang, Y.; Tian, Y.; Song, C.; Wang, J.; Zou, Y.; Anderson, G.J.; Han, J.Y.; et al. A DNA nanorobot functions as a cancer therapeutic in response to a molecular trigger in vivo. *Nat. Biotechnol.* **2018**, *36*, 258–264. [CrossRef]
3. Cho, K.; Wang, X.; Nie, S.; Chen, Z.; Shin, D.M. Therapeutic Nanoparticles for Drug Delivery in Cancer. *Clin. Cancer Res.* **2008**, *14*, 1310. [CrossRef]
4. Goel, S.; Ferreira, C.A.; Chen, F.; Ellison, P.A.; Siamof, C.M.; Barnhart, T.E.; Cai, W. Activatable Hybrid Nanotheranostics for Tetramodal Imaging and Synergistic Photothermal/Photodynamic Therapy. *Adv. Mater.* **2018**, *30*, 1704367. [CrossRef]
5. Wang, H.; Agarwal, P.; Zhao, G.; Ji, G.; Jewell, C.M.; Fisher, J.P.; Lu, X.; He, X. Overcoming Ovarian Cancer Drug Resistance with a Cold Responsive Nanomaterial. *ACS Cent. Sci.* **2018**, *4*, 567–581. [CrossRef]
6. Zhu, Y.X.; Jia, H.R.; Pan, G.Y.; Ulrich, N.W.; Chen, Z.; Wu, F.G. Development of a Light-Controlled Nanoplatform for Direct Nuclear Delivery of Molecular and Nanoscale Materials. *J. Am. Chem. Soc.* **2018**, *140*, 4062–4070. [CrossRef]
7. Wuttke, S.; Lismont, M.; Escudero, A.; Rungtaweevoranit, B.; Parak, W.J. Positioning metal-organic framework nanoparticles within the context of drug delivery—A comparison with mesoporous silica nanoparticles and dendrimers. *Biomaterials* **2017**, *123*, 172–183. [CrossRef]

8. Chen, W.; Wu, C. Synthesis, functionalization, and applications of metal–organic frameworks in biomedicine. *Dalton Trans.* **2018**, *47*, 2114–2133. [CrossRef] [PubMed]
9. Kirchon, A.; Feng, L.; Drake, H.F.; Joseph, E.A.; Zhou, H.C. From fundamentals to applications: A toolbox for robust and multifunctional MOF materials. *Chem. Soc. Rev.* **2018**, *47*, 8611–8638. [CrossRef] [PubMed]
10. Kitagawa, S.; Kitaura, R.; Noro, S. Functional Porous Coordination Polymers. *Angew. Chem. Int. Ed.* **2004**, *43*, 2334–2375. [CrossRef] [PubMed]
11. Lee, J.; Farha, O.K.; Roberts, J.; Scheidt, K.A.; Nguyen, S.T.; Hupp, J.T. Metal–organic framework materials as catalysts. *Chem. Soc. Rev.* **2009**, *38*, 1450–1459. [CrossRef]
12. Liu, Y.; Zhao, Y.; Chen, X. Bioengineering of Metal-organic Frameworks for Nanomedicine. *Theranostics* **2019**, *9*, 3122–3133. [CrossRef]
13. Dong, Z.; Sun, Y.; Chu, J.; Zhang, X.; Deng, H. Multivariate Metal–Organic Frameworks for Dialing-in the Binding and Programming the Release of Drug Molecules. *J. Am. Chem. Soc.* **2017**, *139*, 14209–14216. [CrossRef]
14. Chen, Y.; Li, P.; Modica, J.A.; Drout, R.J.; Farha, O.K. Acid-Resistant Mesoporous Metal–Organic Framework toward Oral Insulin Delivery: Protein Encapsulation, Protection, and Release. *J. Am. Chem. Soc.* **2018**, *140*, 5678–5681. [CrossRef]
15. Wu, Q.; Niu, M.; Chen, X.; Tan, L.; Fu, C.; Ren, X.; Ren, J.; Li, L.; Xu, K.; Zhong, H.; et al. Biocompatible and biodegradable zeolitic imidazolate framework/polydopamine nanocarriers for dual stimulus triggered tumor thermo-chemotherapy. *Biomaterials* **2018**, *162*, 132–143. [CrossRef]
16. Yuan, S.; Feng, L.; Wang, K.; Pang, J.; Bosch, M.; Lollar, C.; Sun, Y.; Qin, J.; Yang, X.; Zhang, P.; et al. Stable Metal–Organic Frameworks: Design, Synthesis, and Applications. *Adv. Mater.* **2018**, *30*, e1704303. [CrossRef]
17. He, C.; Liu, D.; Lin, W. Nanomedicine Applications of Hybrid Nanomaterials Built from Metal–Ligand Coordination Bonds: Nanoscale Metal–Organic Frameworks and Nanoscale Coordination Polymers. *Chem. Rev.* **2015**, *115*, 11079–11108. [CrossRef]
18. Prabhakar, U.; Maeda, H.; Jain, R.K.; Sevick-Muraca, E.M.; Zamboni, W.; Farokhzad, O.C.; Barry, S.T.; Gabizon, A.; Grodzinski, P.; Blakey, D.C. Challenges and key considerations of the enhanced permeability and retention effect for nanomedicine drug delivery in oncology. *Cancer Res.* **2013**, *73*, 2412–2417. [CrossRef]
19. Wang, X.G.; Xu, L.; Li, M.J.; Zhang, X.Z. Construction of Flexible-on-Rigid Hybrid-Phase Metal–Organic Frameworks for Controllable Multi-Drug Delivery. *Angew. Chem. Int. Ed.* **2020**, *59*, 18078–18086. [CrossRef] [PubMed]
20. Chen, Y.; Li, Z.H.; Pan, P.; Hu, J.J.; Cheng, S.X.; Zhang, X.Z. Tumor-Microenvironment-Triggered Ion Exchange of a Metal–Organic Framework Hybrid for Multimodal Imaging and Synergistic Therapy of Tumors. *Adv. Mater.* **2020**, *32*, e2001452. [CrossRef] [PubMed]
21. Peng, S.; Bie, B.; Sun, Y.; Liu, M.; Cong, H.; Zhou, W.; Xia, Y.; Tang, H.; Deng, H.; Zhou, X. Metal-organic frameworks for precise inclusion of single-stranded DNA and transfection in immune cells. *Nat. Commun.* **2018**, *9*, 1293. [CrossRef]
22. Lu, K.; He, C.; Lin, W. Nanoscale metal–organic framework for highly effective photodynamic therapy of resistant head and neck cancer. *J. Am. Chem. Soc.* **2014**, *136*, 16712–16715. [CrossRef]
23. Lu, K.; He, C.; Lin, W. A Chlorin-Based Nanoscale Metal–Organic Framework for Photodynamic Therapy of Colon Cancers. *J. Am. Chem. Soc.* **2015**, *137*, 7600–7603. [CrossRef]
24. Roder, R.; Preiss, T.; Hirschle, P.; Steinborn, B.; Zimpel, A.; Hohn, M.; Radler, J.O.; Bein, T.; Wagner, E.; Wuttke, S.; et al. Multifunctional Nanoparticles by Coordinative Self-Assembly of His-Tagged Units with Metal–Organic Frameworks. *J. Am. Chem. Soc.* **2017**, *139*, 2359–2368. [CrossRef]
25. Alsaiari, S.K.; Patil, S.; Alyami, M.; Alamoudi, K.O.; Aleisa, F.A.; Merzaban, J.S.; Li, M.; Khashab, N.M. Endosomal Escape and Delivery of CRISPR/Cas9 Genome Editing Machinery Enabled by Nanoscale Zeolitic Imidazolate Framework. *J. Am. Chem. Soc.* **2017**, *140*, 143–146. [CrossRef]
26. Zhao, M.; Yuan, K.; Wang, Y.; Li, G.; Guo, J.; Gu, L.; Hu, W.; Zhao, H.; Tang, Z. Metal–organic frameworks as selectivity regulators for hydrogenation reactions. *Nature* **2016**, *539*, 76–80. [CrossRef]
27. Horcajada, P.; Chalati, T.; Serre, C.; Gillet, B.; Sebrie, C.; Baati, T.; Eubank, J.F.; Heurtaux, D.; Clayette, P.; Kreuz, C.; et al. Porous metal–organic-framework nanoscale carriers as a potential platform for drug delivery and imaging. *Nat. Mater.* **2009**, *9*, 172–178. [CrossRef]
28. Zheng, H.; Zhang, Y.; Liu, L.; Wan, W.; Guo, P.; Nystrom, A.M.; Zou, X. One-pot Synthesis of Metal–Organic Frameworks with Encapsulated Target Molecules and Their Applications for Controlled Drug Delivery. *J. Am. Chem. Soc.* **2016**, *138*, 962–968. [CrossRef]
29. Wan, S.-S.; Cheng, Q.; Zeng, X.; Zhang, X.-Z. A Mn(III)-Sealed Metal–Organic Framework Nanosystem for Redox-Unlocked Tumor Theranostics. *ACS Nano* **2019**, *13*, 6561–6571. [CrossRef]
30. Zeng, J.-Y.; Zhang, M.-K.; Peng, M.-Y.; Gong, D.; Zhang, X.-Z. Porphyrinic Metal-Organic Frameworks Coated Gold Nanorods as a Versatile Nanoplatform for Combined Photodynamic/Photothermal/Chemotherapy of Tumor. *Adv. Funct. Mater.* **2018**, *28*, 1705451. [CrossRef]
31. He, Z.; Dai, Y.; Li, X.; Guo, D.; Liu, Y.; Huang, X.; Jiang, J.; Wang, S.; Zhu, G.; Zhang, F.; et al. Hybrid Nanomedicine Fabricated from Photosensitizer-Terminated Metal-Organic Framework Nanoparticles for Photodynamic Therapy and Hypoxia-Activated Cascade Chemotherapy. *Small* **2019**, *15*, e1804131. [CrossRef]
32. Yang, C.; Chen, K.; Chen, M.; Hu, X.; Huan, S.-Y.; Chen, L.; Song, G.; Zhang, X.-B. Nanoscale Metal–Organic Framework Based Two-Photon Sensing Platform for Bioimaging in Live Tissue. *Anal. Chem.* **2019**, *91*, 2727–2733. [CrossRef]

33. Zhang, K.; Yu, Z.; Meng, X.; Zhao, W.; Shi, Z.; Yang, Z.; Dong, H.; Zhang, X. A Bacteriochlorin-Based Metal–Organic Framework Nanosheet Superoxide Radical Generator for Photoacoustic Imaging-Guided Highly Efficient Photodynamic Therapy. *Adv. Sci.* **2019**, *6*, 1900530. [CrossRef]
34. Yin, S.-Y.; Song, G.; Yang, Y.; Zhao, Y.; Wang, P.; Zhu, L.-M.; Yin, X.; Zhang, X.-B. Persistent Regulation of Tumor Microenvironment via Circulating Catalysis of MnFe2O4@Metal–Organic Frameworks for Enhanced Photodynamic Therapy. *Adv. Funct. Mater.* **2019**, *29*, 1901417. [CrossRef]
35. Zhang, D.; Ye, Z.; Wei, L.; Luo, H.; Xiao, L. Cell Membrane-Coated Porphyrin Metal–Organic Frameworks for Cancer Cell Targeting and O2-Evolving Photodynamic Therapy. *ACS Appl. Mater. Interfaces* **2019**, *11*, 39594–39602. [CrossRef]
36. Tian, X.-T.; Cao, P.-P.; Zhang, H.; Li, Y.-H.; Yin, X.-B. GSH-activated MRI-guided enhanced photodynamic- and chemo-combination therapy with a MnO2-coated porphyrin metal organic framework. *Chem. Commun.* **2019**, *55*, 6241–6244. [CrossRef]
37. Liu, M.; Wang, L.; Zheng, X.; Liu, S.; Xie, Z. Hypoxia-Triggered Nanoscale Metal–Organic Frameworks for Enhanced Anticancer Activity. *ACS Appl. Mater. Interfaces* **2018**, *10*, 24638–24647. [CrossRef]
38. Liu, J.; Yang, G.; Zhu, W.; Dong, Z.; Yang, Y.; Chao, Y.; Liu, Z. Light-controlled drug release from singlet-oxygen sensitive nanoscale coordination polymers enabling cancer combination therapy. *Biomaterials* **2017**, *146*, 40–48. [CrossRef]
39. Robison, L.; Zhang, L.; Drout, R.J.; Li, P.; Haney, C.R.; Brikha, A.; Noh, H.; Mehdi, B.L.; Browning, N.D.; Dravid, V.P.; et al. A Bismuth Metal–Organic Framework as a Contrast Agent for X-ray Computed Tomography. *ACS Appl. Bio Mater.* **2019**, *2*, 1197–1203. [CrossRef]
40. Hu, X.; Lu, Y.; Zhou, L.; Chen, L.; Yao, T.; Liang, S.; Han, J.; Dong, C.; Shi, S. Post-synthesis strategy to integrate porphyrinic metal–organic frameworks with CuS NPs for synergistic enhanced photo-therapy. *J. Mater. Chem. B* **2020**, *8*, 935–944. [CrossRef]
41. Li, B.; Wang, X.; Chen, L.; Zhou, Y.; Dang, W.; Chang, J.; Wu, C. Ultrathin Cu-TCPP MOF nanosheets: A new theragnostic nanoplatform with magnetic resonance/near-infrared thermal imaging for synergistic phototherapy of cancers. *Theranostics* **2018**, *8*, 4086–4096. [CrossRef] [PubMed]
42. Zhang, Z.; Sang, W.; Xie, L.; Dai, Y. Metal-organic frameworks for multimodal bioimaging and synergistic cancer chemotherapy. *Coord. Chem. Rev.* **2019**, *399*, 213022. [CrossRef]
43. Chowdhury, M.A. Metal-Organic-Frameworks as Contrast Agents in Magnetic Resonance Imaging. *ChemBioEng Rev.* **2017**, *4*, 225–239. [CrossRef]
44. Della Rocca, J.; Liu, D.; Lin, W. Nanoscale Metal–Organic Frameworks for Biomedical Imaging and Drug Delivery. *Accounts Chem. Res.* **2011**, *44*, 957–968. [CrossRef]
45. Chen, D.; Yang, D.; Dougherty, C.A.; Lu, W.; Wu, H.; He, X.; Cai, T.; Van Dort, M.E.; Ross, B.D.; Hong, H. In Vivo Targeting and Positron Emission Tomography Imaging of Tumor with Intrinsically Radioactive Metal–Organic Frameworks Nanomaterials. *ACS Nano* **2017**, *11*, 4315–4327. [CrossRef]
46. Zhang, K.; Meng, X.; Cao, Y.; Yang, Z.; Dong, H.; Zhang, Y.; Lu, H.; Shi, Z.; Zhang, X. Metal-Organic Framework Nanoshuttle for Synergistic Photodynamic and Low-Temperature Photothermal Therapy. *Adv. Funct. Mater.* **2018**, *28*, 1804634. [CrossRef]
47. Qin, Y.-T.; Peng, H.; He, X.-W.; Li, W.-Y.; Zhang, Y.-K. pH-Responsive Polymer-Stabilized ZIF-8 Nanocomposites for Fluorescence and Magnetic Resonance Dual-Modal Imaging-Guided Chemo-/Photodynamic Combinational Cancer Therapy. *ACS Appl. Mater. Interfaces* **2019**, *11*, 34268–34281. [CrossRef] [PubMed]
48. Wang, Y.; Pang, Y.; Wang, J.; Cheng, Y.; Song, Y.; Sun, Q.; You, Q.; Tan, F.; Li, J.; Li, N. Magnetically-targeted and near infrared fluorescence/magnetic resonance/photoacoustic imaging-guided combinational anti-tumor phototherapy based on polydopamine-capped magnetic Prussian blue nanoparticles. *J. Mater. Chem. B* **2018**, *6*, 2460–2473. [CrossRef]
49. Du, T.; Zhao, C.; ur Rehman, F.; Lai, L.; Li, X.; Sun, Y.; Luo, S.; Jiang, H.; Gu, N.; Selke, M.; et al. In Situ Multimodality Imaging of Cancerous Cells Based on a Selective Performance of Fe2+-Adsorbed Zeolitic Imidazolate Framework-8. *Adv. Funct. Mater.* **2016**, *27*, 1603926. [CrossRef]
50. Shang, W.; Zeng, C.; Du, Y.; Hui, H.; Liang, X.; Chi, C.; Wang, K.; Wang, Z.; Tian, J. Core-Shell Gold Nanorod@Metal–Organic Framework Nanoprobes for Multimodality Diagnosis of Glioma. *Adv. Mater.* **2017**, *29*, 1604381. [CrossRef]
51. Cai, W.; Gao, H.; Chu, C.; Wang, X.; Wang, J.; Zhang, P.; Lin, G.; Li, W.; Liu, G.; Chen, X. Engineering Phototheranostic Nanoscale Metal–Organic Frameworks for Multimodal Imaging-Guided Cancer Therapy. *ACS Appl. Mater. Interfaces* **2017**, *9*, 2040–2051. [CrossRef] [PubMed]
52. Zhang, H.; Shang, Y.; Li, Y.-H.; Sun, S.-K.; Yin, X.-B. Smart Metal–Organic Framework-Based Nanoplatforms for Imaging-Guided Precise Chemotherapy. *ACS Appl. Mater. Interfaces* **2019**, *11*, 1886–1895. [CrossRef]
53. Liu, J.; Yang, Y.; Zhu, W.; Yi, X.; Dong, Z.; Xu, X.; Chen, M.; Yang, K.; Lu, G.; Jiang, L.; et al. Nanoscale metal−organic frameworks for combined photodynamic & radiation therapy in cancer treatment. *Biomaterials* **2016**, *97*, 1–9. [CrossRef] [PubMed]
54. Ni, K.; Aung, T.; Li, S.; Fatuzzo, N.; Liang, X.; Lin, W. Nanoscale Metal-Organic Framework Mediates Radical Therapy to Enhance Cancer Immunotherapy. *Chem* **2019**, *5*, 1892–1913. [CrossRef]
55. Fu, C.; Zhou, H.; Tan, L.; Huang, Z.; Wu, Q.; Ren, X.; Ren, J.; Meng, X. Microwave-Activated Mn-Doped Zirconium Metal–Organic Framework Nanocubes for Highly Effective Combination of Microwave Dynamic and Thermal Therapies Against Cancer. *ACS Nano* **2018**, *12*, 2201–2210. [CrossRef]
56. Lan, G.; Ni, K.; Veroneau, S.S.; Song, Y.; Lin, W. Nanoscale Metal–Organic Layers for Radiotherapy–Radiodynamic Therapy. *J. Am. Chem. Soc.* **2018**, *140*, 16971–16975. [CrossRef]

57. Horcajada, P.; Serre, C.; Vallet-Regi, M.; Sebban, M.; Taulelle, F.; Ferey, G. Metal–organic frameworks as efficient materials for drug delivery. *Angew. Chem. Int. Ed.* **2006**, *45*, 5974–5978. [CrossRef]
58. Gao, S.; Zheng, P.; Li, Z.; Feng, X.; Yan, W.; Chen, S.; Guo, W.; Liu, D.; Yang, X.; Wang, S.; et al. Biomimetic O2-Evolving metal-organic framework nanoplatform for highly efficient photodynamic therapy against hypoxic tumor. *Biomaterials* **2018**, *178*, 83–94. [CrossRef]
59. Ling, D.; Li, H.; Xi, W.; Wang, Z.; Bednarkiewicz, A.; Dibaba, S.T.; Shi, L.; Sun, L. Heterodimers made of metal–organic frameworks and upconversion nanoparticles for bioimaging and pH-responsive dual-drug delivery. *J. Mater. Chem. B* **2020**, *8*, 1316–1325. [CrossRef]
60. Meng, X.; Deng, J.; Liu, F.; Guo, T.; Liu, M.; Dai, P.; Fan, A.; Wang, Z.; Zhao, Y. Triggered All-Active Metal Organic Framework: Ferroptosis Machinery Contributes to the Apoptotic Photodynamic Antitumor Therapy. *Nano Lett.* **2019**, *19*, 7866–7876. [CrossRef]
61. Zhang, L.; Li, S.; Chen, X.; Wang, T.; Li, L.; Su, Z.; Wang, C. Tailored Surfaces on 2D Material: UFO-Like Cyclodextrin-Pd Nanosheet/Metal Organic Framework Janus Nanoparticles for Synergistic Cancer Therapy. *Adv. Funct. Mater.* **2018**, *28*, 1803815. [CrossRef]
62. Zheng, D.-W.; Lei, Q.; Zhu, J.-Y.; Fan, J.-X.; Li, C.-X.; Li, C.; Xu, Z.; Cheng, S.-X.; Zhang, X.-Z. Switching Apoptosis to Ferroptosis: Metal–Organic Network for High-Efficiency Anticancer Therapy. *Nano Lett.* **2017**, *17*, 284–291. [CrossRef]
63. Zhang, Y.; Lin, L.; Liu, L.; Liu, F.; Sheng, S.; Tian, H.; Chen, X. Positive feedback nanoamplifier responded to tumor microenvironments for self-enhanced tumor imaging and therapy. *Biomaterials* **2019**, *216*, 119255. [CrossRef] [PubMed]
64. Li, Y.; Zhang, K.; Liu, P.; Chen, M.; Zhong, Y.; Ye, Q.; Wei, M.Q.; Zhao, H.; Tang, Z. Encapsulation of Plasmid DNA by Nanoscale Metal–Organic Frameworks for Efficient Gene Transportation and Expression. *Adv. Mater.* **2019**, *31*, e1901570. [CrossRef] [PubMed]
65. Alyami, M.Z.; Alsaiari, S.K.; Li, Y.; Qutub, S.S.; Aleisa, F.A.; Sougrat, R.; Merzaban, J.S.; Khashab, N.M. Cell-Type-Specific CRISPR/Cas9 Delivery by Biomimetic Metal Organic Frameworks. *J. Am. Chem. Soc.* **2020**, *142*, 1715–1720. [CrossRef]
66. Du, T.; Qin, Z.; Zheng, Y.; Jiang, H.; Weizmann, Y.; Wang, X. The "Framework Exchange"-Strategy-Based MOF Platform for Biodegradable Multimodal Therapy. *Chem* **2019**, *5*, 2942–2954. [CrossRef]
67. He, Y.; Huang, X.; Wang, C.; Li, X.; Liu, Y.; Zhou, Z.; Wang, S.; Zhang, F.; Wang, Z.; Jacobson, O.; et al. A Catalase-Like Metal-Organic Framework Nanohybrid for O2-Evolving Synergistic Chemoradiotherapy. *Angew. Chem. Int. Ed.* **2019**, *58*, 8752–8756. [CrossRef]
68. Liu, J.; Liu, T.; Du, P.; Zhang, L.; Lei, J. Metal–Organic Framework (MOF) Hybrid as a Tandem Catalyst for Enhanced Therapy against Hypoxic Tumor Cells. *Angew. Chem. Int. Ed.* **2019**, *58*, 7808–7812. [CrossRef]
69. Ni, K.; Lan, G.; Veroneau, S.S.; Duan, X.; Song, Y.; Lin, W. Nanoscale metal-organic frameworks for mitochondria-targeted radiotherapy-radiodynamic therapy. *Nat. Commun.* **2018**, *9*, 4321. [CrossRef]
70. Yang, P.; Men, Y.; Tian, Y.; Cao, Y.; Zhang, L.; Yao, X.; Yang, W. Metal–Organic Framework Nanoparticles with Near-Infrared Dye for Multimodal Imaging and Guided Phototherapy. *ACS Appl. Mater. Interfaces* **2019**, *11*, 11209–11219. [CrossRef]
71. Giménez-Marqués, M.; Hidalgo, T.; Serre, C.; Horcajada, P. Nanostructured metal–organic frameworks and their bio-related applications. *Coord. Chem. Rev.* **2016**, *307*, 342–360. [CrossRef]
72. Simon-Yarza, T.; Mielcarek, A.; Couvreur, P.; Serre, C. Nanoparticles of Metal-Organic Frameworks: On the Road to In Vivo Efficacy in Biomedicine. *Adv. Mater.* **2018**, *30*, e1707365. [CrossRef] [PubMed]
73. Guo, H.; Yi, S.; Feng, K.; Xia, Y.; Qu, X.; Wan, F.; Chen, L.; Zhang, C. In situ formation of metal organic framework onto gold nanorods/mesoporous silica with functional integration for targeted theranostics. *Chem. Eng. J.* **2021**, *403*, 126432. [CrossRef]
74. Ma, Y.; Chen, L.; Li, X.; Hu, A.; Wang, H.; Zhou, H.; Tian, B.; Dong, J. Rationally Integrating Peptide-induced targeting and multimodal therapies in a dual-shell theranostic platform for orthotopic metastatic spinal tumors. *Biomaterials* **2021**, *275*, 120917. [CrossRef] [PubMed]
75. Zou, M.; Zhao, Y.; Ding, B.; Jiang, F.; Chen, Y.; Ma, P.; Lin, J. NIR-triggered biodegradable MOF-coated upconversion nanoparticles for synergetic chemodynamic/photodynamic therapy with enhanced efficacy. *Inorg. Chem. Front.* **2021**, *8*, 2624–2633. [CrossRef]
76. Meng, X.; Zhang, K.; Yang, F.; Dai, W.; Lu, H.; Dong, H.; Zhang, X. Biodegradable Metal–Organic Frameworks Power DNAzyme for in Vivo Temporal-Spatial Control Fluorescence Imaging of Aberrant MicroRNA and Hypoxic Tumor. *Anal. Chem.* **2020**, *92*, 8333–8339. [CrossRef] [PubMed]
77. Cai, X.; Xie, Z.; Ding, B.; Shao, S.; Liang, S.; Pang, M.; Lin, J. Monodispersed Copper(I)-Based Nano Metal–Organic Framework as a Biodegradable Drug Carrier with Enhanced Photodynamic Therapy Efficacy. *Adv. Sci.* **2019**, *6*, 1900848. [CrossRef]

MDPI
St. Alban-Anlage 66
4052 Basel
Switzerland
Tel. +41 61 683 77 34
Fax +41 61 302 89 18
www.mdpi.com

Biosensors Editorial Office
E-mail: biosensors@mdpi.com
www.mdpi.com/journal/biosensors

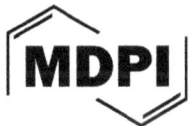